A Long Walk Home

Rachel Clark

With Naomi Jefferies, John Hasler and David Pendleton

Radcliffe Medical Press

Radcliffe Medical Press Ltd
18 Marcham Road
Abingdon
Oxon OX14 1AA
United Kingdom

www.radcliffe-oxford.com
The Radcliffe Medical Press electronic catalogue and online ordering facility.
Direct sales to anywhere in the world.

British Library Cataloguing in Publication Data

A catalogue record for this book is available from the British Library.

ISBN 1 85775 906 0

Typeset by Acorn Bookwork, Salisbury, Wiltshire
Printed and bound by TJ International Ltd, Padstow, Cornwall

Contents

About the author

Rachel Clark was born one of twins, in Charing Cross Hospital, London on 22 June 1970. She and her twin were adopted at birth and grew up with their adopted brother and parents in Bromley, Kent. She was educated at Langley Park School for Girls and at the University of Bristol, where she studied psychology and developed a love of rowing.

Following graduation Rachel trained as an occupational psychologist with Saville and Holdsworth, Surrey, and subsequently worked as a management consultant for Coopers and Lybrand, London. In 1994 she travelled across Asia to take up a two-year secondment in Sydney, Australia.

At the age of 25 Rachel was diagnosed with a rare head and neck cancer. She spent the following three years undergoing extensive cancer treatment, initially in Sydney and then in London. She started to write an account of her treatment and experiences shortly after her return to the UK in July 1996. She lived in Putney with her two kittens Oscar and Ella.

About the contributors

Naomi Jefferies and David Pendleton are occupational psychologists.

John Hasler is a medical practitioner with a background in general practice and medical education.

Acknowledgements

The editors would like to thank Dr Jane Bywater and Mrs Margaret Jefferson for their advice in the preparation of this manuscript for publication.

In recognition of love and friendship, this book is dedicated to Geraldine, Mac, and, most of all, to Sarah.

The names of the doctors and other health staff mentioned in this book have been changed to protect their anonymity and the names of the hospitals have been removed.

Proceeds from the sale of this book are being donated to Help the Hospices and Cancer Research UK.

To Succeed

To laugh often and much;
To win the respect of intelligent people
And the affection of children.
To earn the appreciation of honest critics
And endure the betrayal of false friends,
To appreciate beauty;
To find the best in others;
To leave the world a better place, whereby
a healthy child, a garden patch or
a redeemed social condition,
To know that one life has breathed easier
because you have lived;
This is to have succeeded.

Ralph Waldo-Emerson

Introduction – orienteering and oncology

Naomi Jefferies

'Navigating your way through cancer and its treatment is rather like being dropped in a strange city, without a map or a compass. There are no landmarks that you recognise and no familiar features. This city has no signs, no one speaks your language and your requests for help are incomprehensible: they are unable to help you.'

These words began Rachel's account of her experiences as she underwent the diagnosis and treatment of cancer. Although her particular form of cancer was rare, her emotions and experiences of healthcare were not unusual. Indeed, they mirror those of many people, both those with cancer and those with other conditions.

This book documents her story and spells out important messages for patients and the health professionals who look after them. It is, in essence, about the communication and relationships between these groups of people. Her tale is powerful and evocative – a young person's fight with cancer. However, she is also able to stand back from the fears and frustrations of living with malignant disease, and make sense of her experiences from a wider perspective. It is this ability to recount her poignant observations, sometimes with humour and always with a view to providing learning opportunities for health professionals, that makes this text so valuable.

Dr John Hasler and Dr David Pendleton have drawn out some of these learning points from Rachel's story in an effort to underline that effective healthcare is patient-centred in every sense.

CHAPTER 1

Inside out and upside down – diagnosis

I could feel it everywhere. I inhaled its smell, let its tastes run across my tongue, its sounds echo in my ears. I could sense its warmth spreading across the city, a smooth and golden treacle flowing through the streets, over buildings and houses, and onwards into the sea. A brilliant sun scorched the jacaranda trees which showered the city with a confetti of gentle purple flowers. Blue skies reflected in the harbour's mirror as it sparkled and glistened like liquid diamonds. The eye could skim across its gleaming surface and climbing, continue up and up to the pinnacle of the skyline. The skyscrapers shone, radiating beads of a harder light, scattering beams in random directions as the piercing rays reflected off the thousands of symmetrical windowpanes. Rows and columns of the city's transparent mask. The mask of Sydney, as it welcomed the summer.

I too, as the city, was melting into summer. Indulgently I sucked in its heat through every pore. With growing anticipation I awaited its promises of mornings at the beach merging into balmy days and evenings at streetside cafés. Sunny days, days full of friends and fun, games of tennis, swimming in the sea. Days to fill with my own idealistic hopes, dreams and plans. My life was good and deep down I knew it. I lived in a characteristic terraced house in the city's leafy eastern suburbs, sharing with two wonderful girlfriends and a big red cat. We had a warm and welcoming home that was, more often than not, full of friends and laughter. I had a good job with an international company and, at my own request, I had been granted my dream secondment from London – two years in Australia. I had made a colourful group of interesting and enjoyable friends, I had the time to do the sport and exercise I loved, my life was full of new adventures and opportunities. Everything seemed rosy to me. Nothing in my experiences could have led me to imagine, even in my wildest dreams, the challenges that lay ahead of me. Could anything have prepared me for the biggest, highest, widest hurdle of my life? I was 25 years old. I was diagnosed with cancer.

Hindsight reminds me that there were some 'warning symptoms', but hindsight is, of course, a wonderful thing. Nothing I was experiencing appeared to me to be particularly out of the ordinary. I'd been pretty tired for a while but I had all the explanations. I had just moved house, there had been a few hiccups in my personal life, and, of course, there was that constant sinusitis that was proving so difficult to shift. It must, I reasoned, be the combination of several minor events that were getting on top of me. I had paid a number of visits to a GP culminating in a vast array of antibiotics and nasal sprays. I was on great terms with the local pharmacist, probably stocking a greater range of medications in my medicine cabinet than he did on his tower of shelves. My GP was beginning to despair of me.

'Maybe you're allergic to Sydney,' he suggested unhelpfully, 'maybe you should consider moving.' Regarding this advice as impractical, I tried a different GP. He again tried a further range of pills and sprays to no avail. 'One of my friends with awful sinuses tried squirting garlic oil up his nose,' he tried in desperation, 'you could always try that.'

He began an elaborate description of how his friend had constructed his personal garlic spray, but, sensing my rather lukewarm response, trailed off, deciding not to pursue his line of discussion any further. I did not know what to try. My own rather simplistic 'leave it and it'll go away' approach appeared to have as little validity as my GP's garlic oil. I had to find something. Life was becoming a struggle. Everything was such hard work. I wasn't strolling through every day in the sun, but jogging, uphill with a full pack, in the rain.

Being visibly below par led my secretary to suggest that I visit her acupuncturist. I decided to try; after all it sounded more feasible than the garlic. The dainty Chinese doctor had a shrunken, wrinkled face, its lines hinting at a lifetime of hidden stories. He was small and silent, he even moved around noiselessly as if he floated above the floor's surface, a soundless hovercraft. My secretary had assured me that he had worked miracles for her. I sat in the waiting room with nervous interest until he ushered me through to a small cubicle containing a doctor's couch covered with a crisp white sheet. He motioned to me to lie down and then, very gently, he placed delicate needles in my hands and face. Tinkly Chinese music echoed in my ears as I peacefully drifted off, sleeping my way through an afternoon that should have been spent industriously at work. I had enjoyed the rest but, overall, I still wasn't any better. Maybe I needed a holiday, just to get away from the pressures of everyday life? I could test out the GP's 'allergy to Sydney' theory and my own suspicion that maybe work stresses were getting to me and that I just needed a break. I successfully discredited both by a sailing trip in the Whitsunday Islands. The day after I returned I was back in my GP's surgery.

'I think I should see a specialist' I blurted out.

I quite surprised myself. I didn't really know what sort of 'specialist' existed, let alone what they would actually be able to do for me. I wondered if I was really making a bit too much fuss over the whole thing.

Two weeks later I was sitting in a chair in a Macquarie Street (Sydney's version of Harley Street) consulting room. It was a fairly small room, well filled by dark, old style wooden furniture. The ear, nose and throat specialist had peered up my nose through a circular hole in a metal disk attached to a band around his head. What a strange looking instrument, I thought. Seeing little of any note he had anaesthetised my nose with a disgusting tasting anaesthetic spray and then inserted an endoscope (telescopic probe) up my nose. I wriggled in discomfort.

'Hmm' he pondered, 'I can't see much but I had difficulty getting the endoscope through into your sinuses. I think you should have a scan.'

I felt a bit of a sham really. Surely I didn't need to waste people's time by having what I regarded as serious medical attention. I had never had a 'proper' scan before. Dr Haxell seemed a nice man who, we had discovered while I was describing my work to him, was the father of a friend and colleague. I didn't want to bother him with my minor medical concerns. I was sure that he had more important things to deal with.

Fast forward one week. I was back again, in that cluttered consulting room, clutching a large manila folder full of darkly coloured scans. I sat on the edge of my chair trying not to seem impatient, as Dr Haxell carefully studied the scans.

'Well, you're certainly not being neurotic' he said.

I was relieved. At least I wasn't wasting his time being a hypochondriac. He started pointing to the scans, highlighting a light coloured patch that appeared to be an obstruction in the sinus cavities on the right hand side of my face. I learned that sinuses were not just sinuses and that my major blockage was in what was called my ethmoid sinus.

'What is it?' I asked shakily.

'Well, it is probably just a mucocoele or polyps' he said 'although the image looks like it could be a solid mass. It's hard to tell.'

The significance of the latter half of the statement was lost on me as I contemplated the words mucocoele and polyps. Presumably I should know what they meant, I searched my head for definitions but resorted to nodding my head in agreement.

'We'll have to operate.'

His words stopped my searching. Operate. I'd never had an operation in my life. I couldn't think of many friends who'd had operations either. I'd had my teeth taken out under gas when I was nine years old and I'd found that distressing enough. I was surprisingly shaken. I wandered back through the morning sunshine in the general direction of work, immersed so deeply in my own thoughts I could have drowned in them. An operation. I didn't know what to think. I crossed the street in a daze. Not usually a teary person, I was on the verge of crying. I sat in the park trying to pull myself together. I was irritated by my weakness. 'It's just a small operation' I told myself. 'Don't be so pathetic, you can deal with this.' I sat in the sun until the heat of its rays relaxed me and I felt a little more composed before I headed back to work, scans snug in their manila folder underneath my arm.

I had never had many dealings with the medical profession or the medical system before. I had no idea what would or should happen next. Dr Haxell only operated privately but recommended that a colleague of his, Dr Stanton, perform my relatively minor operation. I waited to be given a date. Expecting, through my work in the business world, a fairly rapid response, I was dismayed to discover that Dr Stanton would be unable to operate for another 6–8 weeks. For reasons I don't fully understand, I was convinced that I couldn't wait that long. I was rapidly feeling worse but felt unable to justify so much sick leave. How could I take two months off work to wait for an operation to correct a minor sinus problem? After a tearful phone call to my sister she persuaded me to ring Dr Stanton and explain to him why I felt such an urgent need for attention. Eventually I tracked him down and blurted out my situation. He was, he explained, very busy with conferences, scheduled operations and such like. They were, he pointed out, trying to help me but I would just have to wait. I was obviously irritating him. Something inside me wouldn't accept 'you'll have to wait' for an answer. 'What if I see you privately?' I persisted. He agreed that I could do that and asked me to bring my scans to him between operations at his hospital that week.

So I set off again, manila folder in hand. Dr Stanton found me as a somewhat lost young woman wandering around by the lifts, identifying me by the non-hospital folder of scans. He had, I expect, hoped to allay my fears and concerns for immediate treatment by a quick five minute consultation. A serious faced and mild mannered man, he studied my scans with intense concentration.

'I think you were right to come in, I'll operate on Monday.'

Today was Friday. I would only need to be in hospital overnight, he assured me, it was a minor procedure. 'At least it will all be over soon' I comforted myself internally. Then I would begin to feel better again.

I didn't really have enough time to panic. The weekend was suddenly over. My brother had arrived from England for a year of 'doing Oz' having just graduated from university and in no great hurry to get himself locked into a career and a nine to five routine. Our reunion after a year was only slightly marred by my minor hospital stay looming over the edge of the weekend. For his part, Nick was pleased that he'd get my bed for a day or two rather than the rather battered sofa which was the available alternative, as well as sole use of my car. We drank beer and ate sushi, much to his disgust (the sushi not the beer). It was a welcome distraction to have him around.

Hospital admissions seem to be a slow and complicated process. Within a few hours I'd had a taste of how alienating hospital procedures could be. I sat in my allocated ward feeling very much in everybody's way. The two old ladies in the ward appeared to be part of the furniture. I sat watching them, imagining that I had been transported, an invisible intruder, into a scene from a rather bizarre comedy. Eventually, a disinterested nurse came to ask me some admission questions, then someone else asked me the same things all over again. I'd already begun counting the hours until I could go home. I began to feel quite miserable, until the anaesthetist appeared and life suddenly became more bearable. Dr McCullen, I still remember his name although I only saw him this once, wore bright red socks and a big smile. He was friendly and open, answering lots of my questions and explaining carefully what he was going to do. His questioning over, he disappeared, reappearing again in the operating theatre where he jokingly explained his reasons for being an anaesthetist until I went under. The last thing I remember was laughing with him and one of the surgical nurses. It helped to blunt the edge of my fear.

The first person I remember on coming round was someone by the name of Heather with a pink hat and a white clinical coat. I don't know who she was but she soon faded out of my consciousness, to be replaced, some hours later, by the surgeon's registrar, Dr Reynolds. I was still pretty groggy and my mouth was sore and stiff.

She began to ask how I was feeling. Even before I interrupted her with the expected 'So what did you find?' I knew it was not a mucocoele or polyps, whatever they actually were. Usually optimistic and positive I had a gut feeling that something wasn't right.

'It was a solid mass' she told me.

They had done a biopsy and, when they had the results, they'd be able to let me know what it was. My mouth was sore, she explained, because they'd had to drill through my top jaw, above my right hand incisors, to remove a bung of glue-like mucus. The mass was blocking the connecting passages between the sinuses. I was in no frame of mind to ask questions. I just nodded vaguely and drifted back into a less than comfortable oblivion.

My fit and healthy body stood me in good stead. It had only been a minor procedure and within a week I was up and about and feeling rapidly better. The pressure from my sinuses was noticeably less and I began to believe that, whatever my problem was, 'they', the medical profession, were well on the way to sorting it all out for me. The next step would be the pathology results and then, well, the worst could surely be another minor operation restoring me to my rightful state of, in the belief of most people my age, everlasting health and immortality.

My knowledge of Sydney was still not particularly extensive. I'd been there for a year but really had little concept of a large proportion of the sprawling city. I'd unintentionally restricted my movements to the areas where I worked, lived and visited the still novel beaches. Hopefully requesting directions to Dr Stanton's consulting rooms prompted Sarah, one of my dearest and kindest friends, to offer to accompany me. She was convinced, with some experience of my navigating skills as justification, that I would get horribly lost. She also thought I could do with the company. Independently minded, I would happily have gone alone but learned that day of the value of having support and an extra pair of ears on hand. We still did, duly, get slightly lost but arrived at Dr Stanton's consulting room right on time. Dr Stanton seemed rather rushed and distracted. Maybe his clinic was very full that morning? I was surprised by his manner compared to the kind and helpful man I had met in the hospital. He was reluctant to make eye contact, his manner was strangely awkward and he was hesitant as to where to begin.

'Are the pathology results back?' I asked.

'The preliminary tests have been run and their findings necessitated further tests, I'm afraid.'

'What are they testing for?' Sarah and I asked in unison.

He talked a little more vaguely about the possibilities. I think that he did use the word tumour in this discussion but tumour, to me, meant little more than mucocoele or polyps had meant a few weeks earlier. I was rapidly feeling the need for a medical dictionary or five years at medical school. I asked if he had any idea what the pathology might show.

'One of five things' he replied cryptically, 'three of which we could do something about. Do you have any questions?'

'Yes. Yes' I screamed inside my head. 'I have hundreds of questions. What have I got? What is wrong with me?' Nothing came out.

'When will the pathology results be available?' asked Sarah, taking control of the conversation that I had relinquished. Next week, he thought, but he would be away at a conference. He suggested that we contact Dr Reynolds, his registrar, who would be able to give us the results. My mind was blank as we were hastily ushered out of the room. We'd been in there for less than ten minutes. I was still none the wiser. What was wrong with me? What did I have?

We sat in the car, side by side.

'Sarah, what exactly is a tumour?' my frozen mind began to thaw. 'I mean tumours, they can be all sorts of things can't they, malignant and benign.' She nodded in agreement.

'He'd have said if it was malignant' she comforted.

'But he wouldn't look at us properly' I worried, 'he was so uncomfortable with us.'

'Maybe he just hasn't got good people skills' she countered.

So round and round we went trying to understand the snippets of information that we had been fed. I cried and once I was crying I couldn't stop. Tears of fear mixed with tears of confusion and anxiety, going over again and again the things that Dr Stanton had said, the things that he hadn't said and the way he had acted. I was so grateful that Sarah was able to drive home. I would have been totally incapable of navigating myself to the bottom of my own garden path. The drive home seemed to have grown by miles and miles in the hour since we had made the outward journey.

Dr Reynolds was a young woman, only a few years older than I was. She'd had a pleasant, professional and slightly detached manner during our previous encounter at the hospital. I had rather liked her. As I and my flatmate Emily walked down the hospital corridor to see her we were laughing to ourselves. Two young women laughing about a now long forgotten joke. We were surprised to see Dr Reynolds waiting to greet us, I was already getting used to spending a significant proportion of my time in waiting rooms. She ushered us through to a cluttered consulting room, with too many chairs and a plethora of rather dubious looking medical implements. I recognised some of the ENT instruments from Dr Haxell's rooms. We all sat down and chatted, exchanging social pleasantries for a while.

'So, what did the path. results show? Do you know what it is?' I asked, trying to get down to the issue that had been gnawing at my mind constantly for over a week.

'I don't think it will mean that much to you' she replied.

She sat stiffly in her chair and was obviously ill at ease.

'Now' she continued, 'obviously the first question you will have is how long have you got' she looked directly at me 'and I'm afraid I can't tell you.'

I was confused. What was she talking about? I looked at my friend, her expression was one of equal confusion.

'I'm sorry' I started haltingly, 'I don't understand what you mean. Do you mean how long is it going to take until I'm better? How long the treatment is going to take.'

'No' she hesitated, 'I meant how long have you got to live' she paused 'and I'm afraid I can't tell you that because I'm not an oncologist.'

Here was another medical word I was expected to understand. What was an 'oncologist', and why wasn't one here, whatever they were? I felt more acutely than ever the need for that medical dictionary. A few moments turned into an eternity before she spoke again. 'I have seen these tumours before in children, but never in an adult.' Half-formed questions tumbled around inside my head like washing in a drier, wafting around but never able to get out. I looked up and saw that she was as shaken as I was. How difficult it must be to tell someone who, for all intents and purposes could easily be you, that they have cancer and that you think they are going to die. Hesitantly, I opened the door to the drier in my head. To each poorly articulated question that stumbled out of my mouth she seemed to answer 'I don't know, I'm not an oncologist'; she was right, she wasn't, where was this elusive beast? I asked her to write down the pathology results so that I could telephone Dr Haxell. Maybe he would be able to help me.

'Come back on Monday morning' she told me.

Her parting remark stuck in my mind.

'Please don't go and jump off the Harbour Bridge.'

At least she didn't attempt to tell me to 'have a nice weekend'.

'As much bloody use as a cardboard cut out' Emily muttered as we sat in a traffic jam.

'She didn't know that I didn't know I had cancer' I repeated. 'She didn't know.'

Had I misunderstood Dr Stanton? Had he told me? If he had, both Sarah and I had missed it. He'd mentioned tumour, so this was a serious tumour, malignant. It was cancer. I sat in the Friday night traffic, tears rolling down my face without really noticing. No one was giving me answers. I felt numb. I wished someone would just give me the complete picture. All I knew was that I had some unpronounceable cancer. I wanted information. What did it mean? What was going to happen to me? Was there any treatment? Was I going to die? Someone must know. The tumble drier of my mind had been overloaded. The thoughts were all getting tangled up with each other. It was in danger of blowing up.

We reached home, my safe home, with a newly festive Christmas wreath on the door. It made a stark contrast to the shock and utter helplessness, I had to find out what this all really meant. I sat down and tried to compose myself, to think rationally. I needed information. Could Dr Haxell help me? I hesitated to bother him at the weekend but.... there was nobody else, I was desperate, I had to know what was going on. Forcing myself to stay calm and breathe slowly, I picked up the receiver and dialled.

'I've got something I can't even say' I blurted out as soon as he answered. 'I don't know what it is and they can't seem to tell me.'

I mispronounced my way through the pathology findings while he listened patiently at the other end. He was very calm and kind.

'Why don't you come round for a drink with us' he offered 'and we'll talk about it.'

My flatmates drove me over, they also wanted to know. He welcomed us in and sat us down around the dining room table with a bottle of wine. He proceeded to give us a technical, medical, but clear explanation of my disease. An alveolar rhabdomyosarcoma in my ethmoid sinus (it took me at least two weeks to learn how to say it). He gave us a lot of time to ask questions, however basic they seemed and, most importantly, he gave me hope that a cure was possible. 'Frequent mitosis', he pointed out, meant that although the tumour was growing quickly it would also respond to treatments quickly as they acted on dividing cells. He did not send me off, as the hospital had, to a weekend of extreme anxiety and panic, but gave me sleeping tablets, support and a hug. He responded to my needs as a human being, not as a problematic patient who could be put on hold over the weekend.

That night I called some friends who came straight over. We laughed and talked until the small hours. I washed my sleeping tablets down with champagne. I felt safer with people around me, their normality seemed to cushion me from the very abnormal and unreal situation in which I found myself. I imagined myself drowning in a champagne glass, smothered by the bubbles. I could hardly believe what had happened. Everything felt more and more unreal as I floundered through the weekend. I tried so hard to tell my mother and father calmly and rationally. I felt it was my 'duty' to tell them but I didn't have the information to answer their questions. I didn't want to panic and upset them or want them to be on the next plane out to Australia. I didn't really know what I wanted because I didn't know what I was dealing with. I spoke to my aunt and to my godfather, hoping that they could give my parents some support. I could not deal with my parents' fear as well as my own.

Some people gave me hope, including a family friend in England who was an oncologist. He had little experience of my particular form of cancer, and he hadn't seen my scans, but he thought that my chances should be quite good. 'High cure rates' he had thought. Others buried me deeper in the pit of despair, their own worries piling in mounds on my shoulders, on top of my own. Some had stories of miraculous cures. My sights were focused on Monday, I was marking off time until I could go back to the hospital. Surely then someone would give me some answers.

As I felt myself sinking, support rose up and cradled me from all directions, supporting me as dolphins support their injured companions. Sarah's mother, Geraldine, a highly experienced nurse, drove down to Sydney to come to the hospital with me. A wonderfully warm and sensible person, she was able to offer me practical help and advice. She came round to collect me early because, as she told me, 'I want to tell you some of the things they may tell you in the hospital before we get there, so that I can explain them and they don't shock you.' She talked to me about chemotherapy, about radiotherapy and about removing the tumour surgically. She also outlined some of the side effects. Chemotherapy, should I have it, could make me infertile. I had never questioned my fertility. I had always assumed that when I wanted children I would be able to have them. Then again I had taken many things for granted, including my life. In my work as a 'change management consultant' I had helped businesses assimilate organisational changes. In our own form of jargon we described the condition resulting from an excess of changes as experiencing 'change overload'. At this point people became totally saturated and could not assimilate any more change. I could have applied the label to myself and it would have fitted like a glove. Too many new and strange things were happening to me. How could my life have altered so rapidly? I felt confused and scared, I wasn't really able to process what had happened so far, yet there was so much more to come. How was I going to take it all in?

Dr Stanton was waiting for us at the hospital. Once again he made very little contact with any of us. He was very awkward and uncomfortable, nervously pacing around the room, not sitting. He began to talk us through the scans, glad to have something to focus on other than our faces. He was busily losing himself, and us, in his technical explanations when the door opened and he was interrupted by the arrival of two younger looking men. They were introduced to us as oncologists, so there was one mystery solved for me at least. They spoke together, briefly and inaudibly, my straining ears could pick up nothing. Dr Stanton asked us to leave so that they could discuss my case in more detail. What were they going to say that they didn't want us to hear? We stood in a confused huddle in the corridor, waiting for someone to take control of the situation, a small herd of sheep waiting for a sheep dog. We began walking, desperate for something to do, wandering aimlessly up and down the hospital corridor, the rhythm of our steps counting out the minutes. Eventually, the door reopened and we were hastily ushered back in and seated in a line. Dr Stanton could not have exited more quickly if someone had shouted fire. I felt that in his eyes I was already dead. Maybe he should have taken the measurements for my coffin before he left, to save time later. The radiotherapist followed a close second. We were left with the medical oncologist, Dr Norton. The atmosphere felt much calmer. He sat down and made eye contact with us all. He told us up front that we had as much time as we needed. At last, I thought, someone to answer my questions. He explained that the scans showed a reasonably large tumour in my ethmoid sinus but that they wouldn't be sure of the extent of the disease until they had carried out a range of further tests. Some of the tests that he mentioned I had come across. Others were further foreign medical jargon. They needed bone scans, an MRI scan, a bone marrow biopsy, blood tests, a lumbar puncture to test my spinal fluid and a biopsy of the lump in my neck that I had assumed was a resurgence of my glandular fever. It had not occurred to me that the disease could have spread. I attempted to digest this news. He moved on, explaining the treatment. I would definitely need chemotherapy and, later on, some ray treatment. It was impossible to be specific, he told us, until they had the results of further tests. It was all very well talking about treatment options and further tests but there was one burning question that I had to bring myself to ask.

'You can cure this, can't you?' I looked straight at him.

'Well' he paused, 'we can have a go.'

I needed more than this.

'How likely is it that you can cure this?'

He hesitated, not wanting to go down this avenue of discussion.

'It's hard to put a figure on it, but' he paused 'on a scale of 1–100 it's at the lower end of the scale.'

This conversation seemed unreal to me, as if I was a fly on the wall listening in.

'How low?' I ventured.

'10–25%, depending on the outcome of the tests.'

Sarah squeezed my hand, Geraldine and Emily closed in around me. I don't remember much more about the consultation, just numbness, but when we left I found it difficult to walk. The car seemed to be a long way away.

Someone had just told me that I was probably going to die, and die soon. I looked down at my smooth tanned skin, at the flesh on my arms; these were healthy limbs, this was a healthy body. Other than a tumour my body was fit and well. How could my 'healthy' body just die? What would happen if I died? The world would go on much the same as before but without me. I felt so alive, so here, how could I not exist? It would be, I thought, rather like moving from London to Sydney. The lives of my friends and family in England, of which I had been a part, still went on, but without me. They would all still be here, breathing, walking around, getting on with their lives and I, well I would be somewhere else. I couldn't quite imagine it.

I tried not to be left alone with my thoughts. I was woefully ill-equipped to deal with them. I was in total shock yet trying to deal with questions about my mortality. I took comfort in the people who emerged to support me, my brother, my twin sister, Naomi, who flew up from Adelaide where she was living, the friends around me. Unfortunately, there is only room for one in an MRI machine. Before I was admitted to hospital an outpatient MRI scan (Magnetic Resonance Imaging) was arranged for me. I was accompanied by my wonderful Scottish friend Ralph. Alone with my thoughts for the first time in a claustrophobic tunnel with a great imitation of an earthquake going on around my head was too much for me. I wriggled out of the tunnel and burst into tears.

'What you need is a holiday' the technician advised me. 'I had a holiday last month, went to Bali, made me feel much better about all my problems' which she went on to tell me about in great detail.

'I can't go on holiday, I've got cancer' I told her once she'd finished her chronicle of woes.

'Oh' she said, and disappeared out of the room to summon Ralph.

I would have loved a holiday, a holiday away from the nightmare I had found myself in, but it didn't seem to be high up on my list of possible options. A second attempt at the scan, with headphones and Ralph holding my hand up the tunnel (until the blood supply was totally cut off he tells me, prompting various Billy Connolly jokes) proved more palatable and the scan was completed.

This was to be the beginning of the long line of explorations that my body was required to submit to. Admission to hospital took me away from the familiar and into a totally alien environment. I was no longer the Rachel in my own definition of self, I wasn't the strong and independent person I had thought myself to be, I was Rachel Clark, cancer patient, the girl with the rhabdomyosarcoma. I hated the hospital tags that I felt institutionalised me and robbed me of my individuality. I had a whirl of appointments that I defy any socialite to better. I met the social worker, the nursing team, what felt like an entire rugby side of different registrars and various other medico-types who appeared in my room at random. To each and every person I asked the same question. 'What can I do to help myself get well? What do other people do that works?' I desperately wanted to grasp hold of the situation, to win back some of the control that had been taken away from me. Now I knew what was wrong with me I wanted to be able to fix it. My need for control and understanding increased as my sense of alienation and confusion grew. Every test they wanted to do on me hurt, and each was new and upsetting. The lumbar puncture, taking a sample of my spinal fluid to determine whether the tumour had gone through into the brain, required me to lie flat on my back for 24 hours. That was quickly followed by a bone marrow biopsy in my hip. I knew that this would hurt, it is not possible to anaesthetise bone. I was scared.

'Do lie still. You're making it difficult for me' complained the registrar who was performing the procedure.

'Sorry' I apologised. Difficult for him, how difficult did he think it was for me?

Although I did feel pain I was sedated and, in reality, it was probably more painful for my sister and brother, Naomi and Nick, to watch my fear and discomfort, that is until, they claim, I started talking about brown squiggly worms, at which point I apparently lost their sympathy. It must have been a good sedative.

Regardless of the lumbar puncture I had things to do, or to have done to me, and people to see. My head was pounding and waves of nausea washed over me but I was up and off down into the bowels of the hospital for my bone scans. In an illogical way I believed that total compliance might somehow help me survive. The bone scans were slow and required total stillness. My head was taped to the table to avoid any undesirable movements. I lay there feeling sicker and sicker, counting seconds and willing time to accelerate before I needed to vomit and ruined the scans. Although so obviously necessary, I found these highly technical tests an alienating and isolating experience. What were they? How did they work? I imagined myself as a toy on a factory production line being scanned as a quality check and triggering the faulty goods alarm.

The end of the production line was the biopsy on the lump in my neck. Not high tech, just a long needle. The doctor who took it asked sympathetically which tests I'd been through that day.

'Never mind, this is the last one and it won't take long' he reassured me.

Once it was over I lay exhausted on my hospital bed. I refused to get in it, as if it were an admission of sickness. My head ached so much though, it was good to be flat. I craved the oblivion of sleep. My door opened again and a man put his head around the door. That was my first meeting with Andrew, a medical psychologist working in the cancer area, who was, over the following months, to become a valued guide, support and friend. As a psychologist myself I knew I was experiencing acute anxiety and panic attacks. I would suddenly find it difficult to breathe, as if a tight band was constricting across my chest. It wasn't just my chest constricting but also my mind. I pictured someone heating up a metal headband so that it would just fit over my forehead, and leaving it to cool so that it contracted, squeezing tighter until it could not be removed. Just as they used to make wooden barrels in years gone by, my head had become a barrel, pulled in so tightly that not a thought could escape. I was looking at myself on two levels. Half of me was objectively diagnosing myself, the other half was screaming in blind panic 'But this is happening to me, it's happening to ME.'

I had described my 'barrel' symptoms to Dr Norton, and asked if there was anyone I could talk to. To his credit Dr Norton contacted Andrew. We talked for a while until Dr Norton appeared. At this point Naomi christened him 'Ping'. He had an amazing ability to just pop up, appearing from nowhere, and disappear just as quickly. We almost expected to see a puff of smoke. 'Ping' she muttered under her breath as he happily popped back into the room with his characteristically exuberant energy.

Ping sat down in a chair and chatted to us. After a while he shifted his weight forward in the chair. His manner changed, his face becoming more formal and professional as he began to talk about the test results. Slowly and clearly he told me that the lump in my neck was not, as I had continued desperately to believe, my glandular fever biting back, but that the tumour had spread to the lymph nodes in my neck. My mind started playing with the figures that seemed to be emblazoned across it in indelible ink; 10–25%, surely this so recent news took me down to the 10%. I was angry and upset. I wanted a positive plan for the future, to look forward. A one in four chance was possible, 25% was a manageable figure, but a one in ten, that was nothing. The metal band enclosed around my head, and a further one around my chest. They squeezed and squeezed, forcing out my air, my thoughts, my being. I couldn't breathe, gulping for air as I cried hysterically.

'It's going to be all right' Naomi tried to calm me.

But it wasn't going to be all right. How could it be? I sobbed and sobbed, unable to control my shaking.

'Sorry' I blurted out, between my gulping.

'We've got plenty of time' Ping reassured me. I gradually got control of my breath and tried to focus on the figure sitting in the chair beside me.

'There is some good news as well' he continued, 'the bone scans were clear.'

So the mental calculations began again. What were my chances now? Left alone for a while I continued my hypothetical arithmetic continuously, to be interrupted a few hours later by Ping reappearing with further arbitrary data for my calculation while Naomi was trying to feed me a Thai takeaway for dinner as I lay flat on my back. I was like a baby bird trying to squawk but getting another mouthful of worm every time I opened my beak. Every time I tried to ask a question I got another forkful of stir-fried beef. The bone marrow biopsy and spinal fluid test results were OK.

The following day I was allowed home. I had been in the hospital less than 48 hours but it had felt like a whole other lifetime. I lay flat on my back for several days. The spinal fluid had leaked a little and the headaches persisted for over a week. Every time I put the 'phone down it rang, reverberating through my sore head. The doorbell went constantly. I felt like I was holding court from my bed. So many friends were wanting to do anything they could to help me. I wanted to be able to help myself. Cancer is so terrifying because it is so disempowering. I told the same story over and over again in endless repetition. I joked that I should just leave a recorded message on the answer machine, or make a general handout. In truth it had all got too much for me; the more I repeated the events of the last few days the more real it became. Naomi joined forces with the answer phone to screen calls. Everyone had different advice: dietary changes, Chinese mushrooms, beetroot juice was a big favourite, and even jumping in a particular lagoon with supposedly 'healing properties'. I couldn't concentrate. My mind was full of thoughts about the next step I was facing – chemotherapy.

CHAPTER 2

Ice magic – chemotherapy

My understanding of chemotherapy was, generously speaking, pretty basic. Chemo I presumed meant chemical therapy, but which chemicals and how they got into the body was a mystery. I had no concept of how it worked, and what the side effects might be. All I appreciated was that it could make me infertile. Dr Norton had told me that I would be receiving chemotherapy. The drugs could kill the ova stored in the ovaries, he said. If there was time they could start the IVF program with women (ova can only be frozen fertilised) but time was apparently one thing I did not have. 'Oh well,' I'd replied, trying to make light of such devastating information, 'I can't think of anyone I'd particularly like to have children with.' I needed to know what chemotherapy was before it was done to me.

Throughout my diagnosis I had constantly felt the need for two things, information and reassurance. The reassurance was understandably difficult to give in my current predicament but I really needed the information. I constantly badgered Ping about it. 'Is there any literature about my disease that I could read?' There was little forthcoming. He promised to see what he could find but nothing materialised. On one occasion I clearly remember being told 'you don't need to know that' in answer to my constant questioning. The social worker who was privy to this discussion later told me she'd turned to him afterwards and asked 'How do you know that she didn't need to know that?' My requests were general and non-specific. It was hard for me to know what information I needed. I didn't know what was available. I needed to be guided through it, I was negotiating my way through a maze on a dark night. Such a vast quantity of literature was out there, but what was relevant to me?

I soon found out what chemotherapy was to mean for me. I had a system of three drugs, code named VAC. These would be injected into a saline drip that ran through my veins. The whole process took about two hours and was to become my routine for the following three months. At the outpatients ward I found another saviour who was to help me through my chemotherapy. Guy was an oncology nurse. He was warm, funny and effeminate. He immediately restored me to the status of an individual, distracting me as he took blood samples and tried to find a suitable vein for the drip to attach to. One attempt at finding my veins convinced me that I would be an appalling drug addict. As he injected the drugs through my drip I felt a burning sensation in my veins. The drip made my arm very cold and Guy would get me heat packs to warm me up again. I glanced around the room. Most of the other patients were older people, many wore headscarves or hats to hide their hair. I still could not equate myself with these people and this situation. I knew my hair would fall out, my beautiful, thick, black hair, but it was still intangible, unreal. I couldn't feel what it would be like reaching up and being unable to run my fingers through my hair. To see my face in the mirror without its black and wavy frame. Maybe Dr Norton was wrong, maybe it wouldn't happen to me.

'Will it definitely happen' I had asked him.

'Yes' he had replied cheerfully, 'all your hair will fall out, even your eyebrows. At least you won't have to shave your legs any more.'

He told me that his wife had shaved her hair off and that he hadn't recognised her when she'd come up and kissed him at a party. It was all very well if you chose to do it, I thought, but I was very fond of my hair and hated the idea of losing it. I preferred not to think about it.

As I sat with the drip in my arm Guy would play his current top ten CDs to cheer us up. The drip dripped slowly. I am sure I could have counted the drops. As I sat there the hospital smell and atmosphere permeated my skin, working its way to my core. I stared at the wall and tried to resist it. Once two bags had dripped through I was free to go. I received my drugs on a biweekly cycle. Each time I was sent home with a 'goody bag' containing anti-nausea medication and syringes and vials for the daily injections I needed to have to ensure that my white blood cell count was maintained. These injections were a source of dread for me at first. I had rounded a corner in the outpatients department to see Guy teaching Naomi to inject a hospital pillow. She did not appear to be a natural.

'You're not sticking that thing in my leg' I objected. 'No way.'

Injection time was awful for both of us. It was like driving into an alpine lake. We would dither around on the edge for ages, trying to build up the courage to take the plunge. She didn't want to hurt me and I didn't want to be hurt. Neither of us could relax until we'd performed the daily ritual. After two weeks I sacked my chief injector, much to her relief. A few other friends had a go, with equally as little success. If you want a job done well, I decided, you just have to do it yourself. Once again I started a mental battle with myself.

'It's only an injection. It's quite straight forward.'

'But it's my flesh, I can't stick a needle in myself.'

'You've had plenty of injections, just get on with it, diabetics have to do it for the whole of their lives, this is just three months.'

'It will hurt.'

And so every morning I repeated this drama to myself, it became a ritual. The problem was eventually solved by the arrival of my newly acquired kitten, Molly the Manx. She thought that syringes and vials were great cat toys. My objective became to get the whole thing over and done with as quickly as possible before she got her grubby little paws on my sterile equipment. What had initially been so unthinkable and strange to me eventually became the norm. Get up, have breakfast, brush teeth, inject leg. I was beginning to adapt.

The acquisition of Molly was an attempt to try to deal with the total upheaval in my life. In a matter of weeks I had gone from a hectic work and social life to a life evolving entirely around my home and hospital visits. Molly was company for me, I could talk garbage to her all day. She was so small that she needed lots of love and looking after. It was important to have something to focus on other than myself. Her need for cat biscuits gave me a reason to get up in the mornings. She never asked me about cancer or my treatment once. She still loved me when my hair fell out and would quite contentedly curl around my naked head and lick my scalp. She was a good little friend.

I discussed my initial fears with Andrew. I was worrying about so many things. I was scared of the tumour itself, scared of confronting the fact that I might experience pain, scared that I might die in the near future. I was scared of the side effects of the treatments that I would have to have. I was petrified that I would make the 'wrong' decisions about my treatment, not giving myself the optimal chance of survival. A common theme through our discussion was my fear of not being strong enough to cope with whatever it was that the future would bring. I didn't know what it would bring, but I wasn't convinced that I could deal with whatever the unknown might be. I was scared that the people around me would leave me, that they would not be there to support me the whole way through. I'd always liked to be around people, making close and supportive friendships throughout my life. In this situation I wouldn't have blamed anyone if it was too much to deal with. I would have under-stood anyone wanting to bail out. I rather wanted to bail out myself but that was not, unfortunately, an option. I was desperately scared of coping on my own. Andrew listened to me thoughtfully.

'But you'd still get through it, wouldn't you?' he told me. 'Even if you did have to do it on your own you would get through it, Rachel Clark.'

I paused my worrying to consider what he had said. He was right. There was no other option than to get through it. Other people would be there for help and support but this was my performance, it was part of my journey and I alone could undertake to travel it. I thought back over my life, my childhood experiences. I'd coped with my parents' divorce and the wave of disputed after effects that had rippled through the family. I had coped with the incident of attempted manslaughter on my mother. I had proved to myself that I was able to deal with the things that life had thrown at me. Maybe they were just a practice run to enable me to deal with the biggest challenge of my life. I had no choice but to back myself and believe that I would succeed in managing whatever lay ahead.

'What happens if you're wrong?' Andrew asked me.

He was right. If I backed myself and I was wrong, it wouldn't really matter.

The toxicity of the chemotherapy drugs was beginning to make itself known. I had initially experienced mild nausea but, as the treatment progressed, I felt more tired and more sick. I proved not to be unique and my hair did fall out. I began to moult hair into the shower, all over my pillows, my clothes, everywhere, the house was covered in it. It would not have been a good time to commit a robbery. I would have been very easy to track. There was hair everywhere but on my head. I couldn't stand it. Nick and Naomi's boyfriend, Matt, took me in hand. They installed me on a chair in the back yard with a towel draped around my shoulders. Vidal and Sassoon, as I named them, went to work. With Matt's razor and my ladyshave they split the labour, Nick took the right hand half and Matt the left. Nick was convinced that he had the better result and was really quite impressed with himself. He stood back and admired his handiwork with pride. I rushed and looked in the mirror. The pure round shadow of my head on the ground should have warned me of what I would see. I found myself staring into the eyes of a creature who would not have looked out of place on the set of 'Star Trek'. I was horrified. Before this point I had known I was ill but now I looked ill. I felt that I should have 'I've got cancer' tattooed on my forehead or ring a warning bell like a leper.

Day by day my disease was becoming more obvious and hence more real.

The panic attacks were beginning to lessen as the initial shock wore off but my anxiety was making itself known in other ways. I seldom slept through the night and would sometimes wake myself up crying. The magnitude of what I was facing was becoming evident to me. My mother, understandably concerned, had flown out to Sydney and the usual difficult family dynamics were in play. I was trying to deal with the cancer treatment itself as well as its impact on the people around me. Andrew had given me a useful analogy for dealing with the difficult times in my illness. Discovering that I had been a keen rower he described the disease process as a race. You didn't stop rowing when you got tired but worked to push through the pain barrier, focusing on achieving the final goal, winning. Now I was going for the ultimate goal, my life. It was going to be a long, hard race. I could not just give up trying when things got tough.

I drew an analogy of my own. Months earlier I had been on the island of Lombok in Indonesia and had been climbing a volcano with a friend. It was a long, steep climb, we'd been going for about six hours. The day was scorching, my legs ached and I was exhausted. We were nearing the crater rim where we planned to camp that night when my legs gave up. I slumped into a heap on the ground.

'Let's stop here' I called to my companion, 'it's as good a spot as any.'

He ignored me and carried on climbing.

'Come up here' he yelled from the rim 100 metres up.

'No way' I yelled back, but he wasn't budging. So I got up and started plodding upwards again, muttering and moaning under my breath. My legs were sore, my feet were sore, my body was sore but when I saw it, the beautiful sight from the crater rim, my aches and pains just melted away. Nestled in the basin was a blue lake with clouds of steam swirling upwards. It took my breath away, I would have walked up that mountain all over again if I'd have known what was at the top. That was the picture that I held with me throughout my treatment. For a goal as precious as my life I could expect a very rocky climb but the hardest part would lead to a view that I could only imagine in my dreams.

Fridays were chemo days. Every other week I would drive through the rush hour traffic for the morning of drips, needles and drugs which was guaranteed to write off my weekend. As the treatment progressed I had identified a pattern of how I would feel. The first couple of days following the treatment were the worst. I felt nausea, shivers and extreme tiredness. The symptoms then gradually wore off until I had a couple of days feeling pretty human before it was time for my next hit. Friends began to plan our social activities around my chemo cycle. Weekends away were never planned for 'chemo-weekends', the ones directly following my treatment. I wonder how many diaries my schedule managed to hit? Once, after a treatment, I had burning sensations up and down the veins in my arms where the drugs were injected. In a panic, I called Guy. What was happening? Was it serious?. It was something that sometimes happened, he reassured me, it would go, and it eventually did. On another occasion a fever gave me bizarre body sensations as I lay in my bed. My head felt huge and enormously heavy, my legs were tiny, my trunk long and enlarged. It felt like I was on drugs, it was a scary experience. I didn't want to shut my eyes. I felt very out of control.

Each chemo-Friday I would arrive at the outpatients to have an immediate sample of blood taken. This was whisked off to testing to determine whether I had a sufficiently high count of white blood cells for my drugs to be administered. I would wait anxiously for the result, not wishing to delay and hence prolong my treatment even for a week. This waiting space was partially filled by a consultation with Dr Norton. He would press his fingers into my neck underneath my jaw line, feeling for the lymph node that was a rough and ready guide to how the tumour at the primary site may be responding. I felt that it was decreasing rapidly but Dr Norton never displayed any extreme pleasure or concern over how it was responding. I left each consultation feeling faintly dissatisfied. I felt rushed through, my lack of proactive questioning reflecting my need for someone to help me formulate my questions. When I did articulate my concerns I felt that they were regarded as almost trivial. Maybe they were in relation to some of the concerns that oncologists must deal with, but to me they were critical. My continual badgering for further information was finally answered in the form of a weighty tome, an oncology textbook.

'You won't understand most of it' Dr Norton informed me, guiding me to the appropriate pages. I understood a considerable proportion of the relevant chapter and was grateful to him for arming me with some of the knowledge and understanding that I needed.

CHAPTER 3

Pick'n'mix – alternative therapies and options

My disease had an immediate impact on my daily life in the fact that I was no longer working. What would I do with my days? All that time I would have on my hands. I hadn't realised that having cancer would be a full-time occupation. I burdened myself with guilt that I really should be at work. After all I was just feeling tired and nauseous, I could still manage everyday tasks. I'd asked Dr Norton at the beginning 'Could I still work?'

'Maybe' he'd replied, 'but...' he hesitated.

'You mean that if I've only got a limited time left I probably shouldn't spend it in the office?'

He'd nodded. I didn't mind being at home. It was in fact unusually pleasant. My living room could have been easily mistaken for a florist's shop with the armfuls of flowers that arrived daily from friends all over the world, from colleagues and from clients. I was so touched by the people who wanted to do something for me. But I wanted to do something for myself.

So began my journey into the realms of alternative therapies. The hospital had provided me with some relaxation tapes. I listened to them once and I don't think I ever used them. My constant badgering of hospital staff had elicited the fact that 'being positive' was a good thing. But how positive did I have to be? Was there a positivity scale where a smile might cure a minor cold or skin irritation and a week of belly laughing would combat almost anything?

Neither I nor any of my specialists had any idea why I might have developed this childhood cancer in such an unusual place. If I didn't know the cause how could I find a cure? I began reading. There seemed to be a whole range of different philosophies and approaches I could try. One woman had apparently cured her breast cancer by eating nothing but grapes for ten days (boring, but beats chemo and presumably very good for your fibre intake), a whole variety of conflicting 'cancer diets' were recommended. Psychological factors were also mentioned. I worried that my cancer was due to stress that I had unwittingly put myself under, or that it was related to my somewhat problematic family background. Was I the personality type who was a cancer risk? Was I responsible for my own disease? Had I brought this on myself or was it my family? I was uncomfortable with the idea that there was somebody responsible, someone to blame. Meditation was also recommended as an effective healer. I was hardly the ideal candidate for meditation. How could I meditate, I was far too busy? There are some situations in life when you really are between a rock and a hard place and there was no doubt that I was in one of them. I had nothing to lose and everything to gain by trying all that I could. I wasn't at work, I had plenty of time to devote to discovering the available options. I didn't care how much I ended up in debt, I told myself; after all, what kind of price can you put on your life? Ralph, my Scottish friend, likened it to training for a sport. 'Imagine that you are in training, like when you are rowing. Each day you have to do the things that will help you reach your end goal. In this case it is not running and eating vast quantities of carbohydrates but feeding your body with plenty of vitamins and minerals and doing meditation.' So, with the assistance of friends, I embarked on my voyage of exploration.

A holistic medical centre seemed a reasonable place to start. I was introduced to a doctor who practised meditation. I was open-minded but my less accepting sister described him as 'the one who wanders around being skinny with no shoes'. He took me through some guided meditations fairly similar to the relaxation tapes the hospital had provided. He also gave me a rather foul tasting Indian herb to take with honey. He advised me to meditate twice a day and try to avoid wearing shoes. He suggested that I see the centre's iridologist and naturopath. She confessed that the irises of my eyes, which she studied in great detail, managed to hide the tumour which I admitted to. She prescribed me some slightly less disgusting western herbs and sent me on my way. So my morning ritual extended further to include my herbal potions. Holding my nose to disguise their taste amused Nick greatly.

'It's all a load of crap' he laughed, 'I can't believe you're taking them.'

Undaunted, I continued my quest, organising wonderful massages with pungent smelling oils. I don't know whether the massage helped my disease but it certainly eased my tension. The stresses and strain that were showing in my body could not be good for anybody.

A further yoga practising doctor I visited (this one wore shoes) explained the Indian principles of energy centres, chakras, in the body. His breathing exercises and meditations were based around these energy centres. I was never really sure whether these meditation sessions were effective but something, maybe desperation, made me keep going. I certainly felt much calmer and more relaxed after each one, although I was not particularly supple when it came to sitting in the cross-legged yoga positions. I was regularly brought out of any state of deeper consciousness by the pins and needles prickling in my aching legs. I meditated at home, propping myself up with cushions to avoid cutting off the blood supply to my limbs. It helped me deal with my panic attacks and daily stresses. I reasoned with myself that slowing down my body must create an internal environment conducive to healing. By healthy eating and meditation I tried to help my body deal with the toxic chemicals that were bombarding it.

I was beginning to understand that the Chinese and the Indians had very different approaches to health and life than that espoused by our western model. Having toyed with acupuncture in the past I decided to give it another try. My yoga practising doctor recommended a Chinese doctor in Chinatown. This tall and unassuming man did not speak much English but, apparently, was good with his needles. His treatment system was based on meridians, or energy paths, around the body. His diagnosis consisted of feeling more pulses in the wrist than I knew existed, and carefully inspecting the coating of my tongue. He made careful notes in Chinese characters, and could have been writing his shopping list for all I knew, but my gut feeling was to trust him, that he could help me. He placed needles in my face, arms and legs. Once the needles were in position he would give them a sharp tap. I felt a strange kind of discomfort as he tapped, almost, but not quite, painful, as if energy was being moved around my body. He would leave me for a while and then return to twiddle the needles further, as if he were doing a little fine-tuning. I visited this acupuncturist throughout my chemotherapy. I felt that balancing out my body's energies would help it to deal with the onslaught it was receiving from the chemotherapy.

While I was investigating as many alternative avenues as I could, Dr Haxell was keeping up to date with my progress through the conventional medical system. Unhappy with the radiotherapist I would be seeing, he pushed me to get a second opinion. He had high regard for the team at another Sydney hospital. He encouraged me to take my scans to them and see what they would say. I was reluctant. I had found the whole diagnosis process so shocking and upsetting that I didn't think I could face it all again. Surely any doctor I saw would tell me the same thing, that there was very little hope of a cure. He'd spoken to the doctors at the new hospital and they were expecting me. Sarah agreed with him.

'They're supposed to be very good' she encouraged, 'It won't hurt just to find out.'

So it appeared that I was to get a second opinion. Without a doubt it was the best thing that I could have done.

Naomi, Nick and I found ourselves sitting in a wood panelled waiting room, armed with the manila folder of scans. We were shown through to a consulting room where we sat waiting until, with a great burst of energy, Dr Newbury came flying through the door. I was quite bemused, not really knowing what to make of him. He reminded me slightly of a walrus. We could have been starring in a black version of *Alice in Wonderland*. Dr Newbury was friendly, if slightly abrupt. He sat far too close to me, his face right up close to mine whilst he spoke. He poked and prodded around my head and neck and flicked through my portfolio of scans.

'Hmm' he pondered. 'Can you come back to our head and neck clinic? There are some other people I would like to take a look at these.'

'What are the chances?' Naomi asked 'The other doctor thinks 10–25%.'

'Oh higher than that' he responded, waving his hands in the air, 'maybe 30–40%.'

How could this estimate be different based on the same test results? Oncology appeared, I realised, to be more of an art than a science. Suddenly, Dr Newbury startled me by hugging me hard. Did he think that I was upset? I'd felt relatively calm and together. It seemed a rather inappropriate thing to do. Was he upset himself? Had he been on a training course advocating patient hugging? He had managed, however, to convey to me a sense that this wasn't total disaster and to instil in me, during our discussion, a faith in his professional opinion.

The clinic proved to have both an up side and a down side. It was immensely reassuring to find that a whole team of health professionals from different specialities were looking at my case. The room was packed with surgeons, radiation and medical oncologists, social workers and nurses. I was reassured to know that I was getting a number of expert views. It was, however, alienating to know that a discussion was going on about what was going to happen to my body without hearing the process of their decision making. I was invited in for a brief examination. I was grateful that one of the surgeons had slipped out beforehand to have a quick word.

'We may need to take your eye out' he warned me, 'so don't be shocked if you hear us talking about it.'

My eye for my life, it didn't seem too bad an exchange. The surgeons talked me carefully through my scans. One was particularly gentle and reassuring. I knew that he had been ill himself. Maybe he had an insight of how it felt to be in the patient's seat. They were keen to operate, they told me, convinced that surgery would give me the best chance of survival. Once again the verdict was so different.

I felt my dilemma acutely. I mulled it over and over, discussing it at length with Andrew.

'What were the reasons for each of the decisions?' he asked me. He suggested that I try to interpret the advice from the perspective of the individual doctors in question. What were the key factors driving their decision-making processes? The problem was I wasn't quite sure. The second team strongly advised me to allow them to operate, I would probably lose an eye but at least they could give me some hope. I went back to the first hospital to speak to Dr Norton. Maybe he could clarify the situation for me.

'I do not agree.' He countered the second opinion. 'I believe that major surgery will be traumatic and disfiguring without affecting the outcome.'

So back I went to Dr Newbury, 'Dr Norton is strongly opposed to surgery' I told him.

'Well, it's up to you' he said, 'I'm happy for you to finish your chemotherapy before we operate, but don't leave it too long.'

I had some time to think. The problem was that I didn't understand the criteria for each team's recommendation. How important was the cosmetic factor in their equation? I just wanted the solution that would have the best chances of saving my life. I dragged friends into my quandary. Get a third opinion, they counselled. Put it to a vote and get a majority opinion. Dr Marchant, at a third hospital, was recommended to me, both by a friend who had had cancer and by another friend's medical father. So I fixed an appointment.

Dr Marchant was a godsend to me in a number of ways. He was the first person who spoke to me as an intelligent adult. He was positive and reassuring without sparing me any details or trying to shield me from the severity of the truth. Once again I was sitting as the prime exhibit in a head and neck clinic, but this time I was given an opportunity to ask questions during the session. Dr Marchant and a colleague spent a good deal of time talking me through the clinic discussion and recommendations after the event, patiently answering my own questions and suggesting others that I might like to ask. He was happy to oblige my request for further information about my disease. What sort of information would I like? He elaborated on what was available, suggesting that he ring the city's children's hospital, this being a paediatric cancer, to see if they would treat the tumour any differently. I needed to know that the doctors that I was seeing had looked to other hospitals and other countries to see what was regarded as state of the art treatment for my disease. In the absence of Dr Norton I had once seen one of his colleagues, who had offered to contact hospitals in London and America to see what they would recommend. I had found that very reassuring. I walked out of the consultation with Dr Marchant wondering to myself whether the way that I was acting was affecting the way the doctors were reacting to me. By this point my initial shock was wearing off and I was beginning to handle my own situation more calmly. I had also attended this consultation alone, rather than importing my personal context of friends and family. It was possible, I mused, that this was a more difficult situation for doctors who could identify with me as similar to themselves or their own children. This could explain the reactions I encountered.

Unfortunately, in spite of this positive and helpful consultation, I was no closer to making the decision I had hoped it would help me clarify. The clinic had been split in its opinion. The surgeons believed that my tumour was operable whereas the oncologists felt that chemotherapy and radiotherapy were the preferable treatment options. The following week I returned to find that, true to his word, Dr Marchant had obtained a number of articles and papers that he believed would satisfy my need for information. He was spot on in finding the level of information I needed. Having a psychology degree I was used to reading medical papers. I did not want what I regarded as Mickey Mouse information. Although general information leaflets about cancer were initially useful, I wanted to know specific facts relevant to me. I needed to understand what my disease really was and the range of treatment options available. I did not want to know about outcomes. I realised that previous doctors had been protecting me from the articles that laid out in black and white the limited chances of my survival. However, my basic survival instincts told me that I needed to know what I was fighting before I could formulate my battle plan.

The lack of information that I had previously encountered had prompted a friend to search the Internet. Our limited understanding of which articles were actually relevant to my case was confusing. I waded through the sea of paper he had gathered, trying to work out what was relevant. My understanding of this 'pick 'n' mix' of assorted articles led to the one, and the only one, occasion throughout my illness when I truly believed that I was going to die. That day, Christmas Eve 1995, I was convinced that I would never see another Christmas. To me the future seemed to be a void of never ending nothingness, it no longer existed, I played no part in it. I sat slumped in a chair, in total apathy and despair. There was nothing I could do, no hope, I was surely going to die. I was rescued from my cloying despondency by a call from Dr Haxell inviting me for a drink and Christmas carols. Understanding my anguish he advised that I desist from reading such articles. 'They can be very misleading' he cautioned me. The Christmas carols with their familiarity comforted me. The low evening sun softened, mellowing the contours of the land and with it my mind relaxed. Maybe I could hope to see another year.

At the end of our meeting, Dr Marchant had made me aware of another difficulty facing doctors in treating their patients. We had begun talking about my disease in the present but Dr Marchant had been reluctant to quote any statistics regarding my chances. He was unsure of my chances, he admitted, and was reluctant to mislead me by attempting an estimate. The condition was too rare in adults to have meaningful statistics. Moving on to talk about my future he advised me 'not to think about having a family for a few years'. Having been informed at the outset of my chemotherapy about the fertility risks involved, this was a rather sensitive subject. I did not consider, however, that it was the role of a doctor to advise me on my personal life. Those decisions must surely be based on my own morals and values. The boundaries surrounding such issues are blurry. How difficult to know what sort of advice and guidance would be 'right', and what oversteps the mark. His comment stayed in my mind and I objected to myself 'that's not his business'. I felt mildly angry at him. He'd helped me in so many ways but that final comment had fallen well outside my established boundaries and had resoundingly hit a nerve.

I am not a patient person, yet cancer is a disease that requires, in fact demands, patience. 'How am I doing?' I would ask Dr Norton at each consultation, knowing that the only gauge would be the less than specific lymph node. At last, Dr Norton told me, it was time for another series of scans. We would find out what, if any, effect the chemotherapy was having on my primary tumour. For administrative reasons it appeared to be simplest for me to be admitted to hospital in order to get the scans performed quickly. An appointment was made and Sarah offered to accompany me on the specified date. I was duly admitted and despatched to the CT department. The CT operator was young and chatty. He set up and conducted the scan quickly and efficiently.

'I'll go and see what time your MRI is scheduled' he offered helpfully and bounded off down the corridor. Minutes later he was back.

'They don't seem to know anything about you' he looked confused.

He suggested returning to the ward to try to establish where and when I was expected to be scanned. I was already feeling apprehensive. My stomach was flutteringly reminding me that I had not much enjoyed my previous encounter with an MRI machine. We wandered around the ward looking for assistance, eventually tracking down an absent-minded registrar. He had been 'just about to take the details down' to the MRI department. I deduced, without requiring possession of highly sophisticated detective skills, that booking my scan had somehow been overlooked. He suggested that we return to my room and wait. 'It'll be sometime today, or maybe tomorrow' he told me. I felt a bit of a fraud being given a bed. I didn't need a bed. I just needed a quick scan and then to head off home as soon as I possibly could. We hung around the ward chatting for a while before we lapsed into an aimless flicking through the average selection of out-of-date and dog-eared waiting room magazines. We were startled out of our bored perusing by the arrival of a hospital trolley rolling slowly across our field of vision. The trolley was laden with a body-like shape engulfed completely in a yellow sheet. I stared for a few moments. There was no movement.

'Oh my God' I whispered to Sarah, 'is that a dead person?'

She nodded dumbly. We looked at each other, horrified.

'I'm not staying here' I asserted, 'I'm not that sick.'

I did not feel that I was dying, yet I was sitting in a ward surrounded, or so I felt, by people who were dead or dying. It all began to close in around me. I had to get out.

'Let's go home' I said. 'They can call me and tell me when they know what time the scan is.'

We left.

Twenty minutes later a phone call summoned me back. I drove frantically but the time slot had gone by the time I arrived back.

'You'll have to stay and wait' they told me. 'It'll probably be tomorrow now.'

The idea of spending another night in hospital filled me with horror after what I had just seen. I did not want to be made to feel seriously ill. Every moment I spent there seemed to further complete the transformation from person into cancer patient. I slumped into a chair, too dejected to argue. I sat and stared at the floor, at the walls and then at the ceiling. Minutes seemed to be hours. After I had been blankly observing nothing for some time I was jerked back to reality by a knock on the door. The social worker, Janie, put her head around the door.

'I heard that you were in' she started. 'What are you doing here?' she asked, rather surprised. I told her. And then I carried on telling her – how upset I was by the dead body, how afraid it made me feel, how alienating I found the hospital environment, that I didn't want to be there overnight, that I couldn't understand why the scan hadn't been booked, that I just wanted to leave. I took a breath.

'Why don't you?' she asked.

'Why don't I what?'

'Why don't you just go home?' she suggested. 'You wouldn't normally sit and wait all day for something without any explanation, would you?'

She was right. The whole situation was making me feel totally disempowered. Six months before I would never have just sat in a heap feeling that a situation was totally out of my control. I walked towards the entrance to the wards. I stopped at the front desk and told the sisters and the registrar.

'I'm going home now, I can't stay here any longer.'

As I headed towards the exit the registrar's voice halted me.

'Hold on, I'll just try the MRI department again ...'

Ten minutes later I was encased in the MRI machine's tunnel. Why is it always necessary to be the squeaky wheel? I wondered to myself.

I slept long and deep that night, the strain of the day had exhausted me. Through the haze of my sleep I heard a piercing ring, the phone jarring my mind back into consciousness.

'Hello' I mumbled.

I was greeted by the excited tones of the previous day's registrar.

'There's hardly anything to be seen.'

I was confused, 'Sorry?'

'Your scans' he told me, 'they're markedly different to the originals. The tumour has responded quite significantly to the chemotherapy.'

I should have been surprised, elated, ecstatic. On the surface I was, but something inside of me said 'why are you surprised? I knew it would, I could almost feel it shrinking'. I had always believed that the chemotherapy would cure me. So I had got over my first hurdle, chemotherapy. I may have borne the marks, or lack of marks as far as my hair was concerned, but I'd got through. I turned my attentions to the next step.

Armed with my new scans I set off on my round again. I felt like a travelling salesman touring the hospitals. What did they think of my new range of goods? Both Dr Norton and Dr Marchant's team agreed that I should have an operation. They recommended that I should ask one particular group of surgeons to operate. They were apparently well regarded for their cranio-facial resections. The surprise verdict was from them. The only ones to insist that surgery was essential, the new scans now forced them to reconsider their initial position. The head and neck clinic held a long discussion. They finally emerged to lay down my options to me. Directly they told me:

'Radiation alone will give you a 50% chance of the disease not recurring in the next ten years. Surgery followed by radiation, we believe, will give you a 75% chance. We believe we can save your eye. Which would you like to do?'

I was stunned, not by the options but by the numbers. No one had offered my hopes anywhere near the magnitude of 75% before.

'Well there isn't a choice really, is there?' I told them. 'I have to give myself the best chance I possibly can.' I asked what the surgery would involve.

'You'll end up with a small scar down the side of your nose.' That didn't seem too bad. At least I could keep my eye!

The surgical team would need to wait six weeks for the chemotherapy to work itself through my body sufficiently to withstand a major operation. I had time to myself, time when I actually began to feel better. My skin no longer smelt of chemicals, signs of fluffy baby hair even began appearing on my head. Yet I felt like a prisoner on death row, waiting to hear the date of my operation as if it were an execution date, knowing that it was inevitable. This time allowed me to continue my quest for alternative cures. A work colleague put me in touch with a conventional GP who was also a naturopath. I found myself winding my way up the stairs to her consulting room, wondering quite what to expect. My colleague had simply informed me that she was known to have 'done some good stuff with cancer patients'. Now I was going to find out what that 'stuff' could be.

Dr McCulloch was seated behind a large desk in the corner of the room. I thought her to be in her mid-thirties. She got up to greet me, asking 'So what can I do for you?' She was tiny, and, as I discovered, she certainly had some alternative ideas. She began, as homeopaths do, by asking me about my childhood, about common illnesses and my family. She focused in on an incident when my mother had been attacked and stabbed with a garden fork. She had been injured in her head and in her leg. I had witnessed the incident as a young teenager. Dr McCulloch suggested that as a child, helpless to respond and unable to offer any help in such a situation, I had taken my mother's injuries on myself to try to stop her dying, hence a tumour on the same side of my face as my mother was injured. Plausible? Possible? As yet no one has been able to explain the existence or origin of my tumour satisfactorily so my mind remained open to all possibilities.

She also practised kinesiology. Muscle strength, she maintained, would indicate whether the combination of Chinese herbs she prescribed would suit and help my body. She would put the bottles of herbs on my stomach as I lay on her examining table. She pushed upwards with her fingers underneath my wrist and asked me to resist. Apparently with the correct herbs I would be strong and be able to comply with her request, if the wrong combination was used I would have no strength. I cannot explain it but there were definitely times when, try as I might, I had no strength to resist the equal pressure she applied each time. So my morning ritual expanded further to include Chinese herbs and dandelion tea. She explained to me that the Chinese believed that the meridians, or energy lines, of the body could get blocked and hence cause disease. Chinese treatments often involved balancing the body's energy flows. She suggested that ensuring that all my meridians were unblocked and that tracing the meridian paths, creating a 'blue print' of my energy paths, could help support my body through the trauma it was experiencing. I was willing to give anything a try.

One thing I did not have hard evidence of was that support groups could prolong the life of people with cancer. I interpreted this as an illustration of the mind playing a critical role in determining the outcome of a disease. Bereavement studies show that one can simply lose the will to live. The proportion of partnerships in which one partner dies within a year of their deceased spouse is staggeringly high. It is something that is difficult to understand and impossible to measure. This intangible will to live is effectively our life force. We all have it and we can all tap into it. It is there to be used and I was definitely going to use mine. At first I ummed and ahhed about joining a group. I was fed up with talking about cancer. It seemed like every conversation I had in some way involved cancer. Andrew had to keep reminding me exactly how big my tumour was in relation to the rest of my life, about the size of a golf ball. I was also scared of meeting people who were much sicker than I was. I was scared for two reasons. I didn't want to see what could potentially happen to me. I had to keep seeing myself as a healthy body with a small tumour, not as a 'cancer victim' or any of the other phrases coined by the media to describe people with cancer. I was also worried that I would meet people in a lot of physical and emotional pain and that I would not be able to reach out to them. I might be so tied up in dealing with myself that I would not be able to support other people adequately. So it was with some trepidation that I approached the first of the Tuesday morning support groups, that I eventually began to look forward to.

The groups were held in a yoga room, with chairs and a whole heap of coloured cushions for seating. The setting consisted of two parts, a discussion and a group meditation. We took a blind vote each time about which was to be the first. They were run by a warm and wonderfully serene woman called Jenny, an ex-oncology nurse. She had patience, which I as an impatient person admired, and seemed to have enough time for everybody there. Sometimes the meditations worked well for me but at other times I was mentally writing my 'to do' list, unable to switch off from everyday life. I was a little more successful with my mental discipline at the group than when I was sitting at home alone, listening to a tape. When I gave them the focus they deserved these meditation sessions gave me time to relax my body and give me a calming peace. My turbulent mind was desperately seeking a calm stillness that meditation was sometimes able to give. The group discussions, rather than consisting of the horror stories I had so feared, involved whatever we wanted to talk about. Each week different people were able to contribute something to the others in the group, empathy and understanding, strength, suggestions and tips on how to deal with medical situations and people, practical ideas on alternative approaches and more than anything an open honesty and hope. There was an incredible positiveness in that group, even in those who had secondaries and for whom the doctors believed the outlook was grim. After all, we were all still alive. It was good to have the opportunity to give as well as to get out. To me cancer felt like a burden that engendered my reliance on other people. A heavy load that I could not put down. It was like wearing a backpack on a London tube in the rush hour, accidentally bumping into others at every move and having to be helped off at the right stop. Now I had the opportunity to give just a little something back. That in itself enabled me to feel more of a complete person again. Each week a disparate group of individuals would straggle into that yoga room, and every week would emerge slightly calmer and, I believe, a slightly wiser group of people.

One woman from the group particularly stuck in my mind. Val

was a vivacious person, lively and outgoing. She had a crown of wonderful red, curly hair, chemo curls she informed me, that warmed up her face. She had been diagnosed with breast cancer a couple of years earlier. The doctors had not recognised the tumour earlier, in spite of her insistence that something was wrong. By the time an appropriate diagnosis was made the disease had spread extensively. They gave her very little hope. It would be a matter of weeks they had told her. A 'make sure your will is in order and sort out your affairs' verdict was delivered on her case. But Val had amazing spirit. She and her fiancé had fought her illness all the way. The outlook was grim. Her bones were riddled with cancer. The doctors could not understand why she was even bothering to try to hang on to life. She reported to the group the contents of a letter from one of her doctors to another one which had read 'Why won't Val and her fiancé just accept that she is going to die?' Two years later Val was still very much alive and miraculously cancer free. She experienced a lot of pain while her bones were healing but with indomitable guts she had battled her way through. I couldn't help but feel that those doctors had no concept of what it must be like for someone who loved their life with the zest that Val exuded, to be told that their most precious possession would be so cruelly taken away from them. But of course, I thought to myself, how could they be expected to? Even the most compassionate of people would fail to understand the ferocity with which we humans can cling to life. It is an elusive power that cannot be fully explained or illustrated. Its intensity can only be experienced. As Val had pointed out at one of the group sessions, there are examples of people recovering from every type of cancer at every stage of advancement, long after the doctors have given up hope. There is no clear, generic cut off point where there is no longer a reason for clinging on to life. Some people will give up on hearing their diagnosis whilst others, like Val, will continue on way past their doctors' expectations.

CHAPTER 4

Roots and roses – my origins and image

The diagnosis of my cancer had taken my life and turned it on its head. It was as if I was living in one of those little domes that you can buy in gift shops, the snow scenes with the little plastic houses. I was firmly trapped in a blizzard by some overzealous shaking. Along with dealing with the direct effects of the existence of my cancer and its treatment, I was being forced to adapt my outlook on life. I had to face up to some of the glaringly obvious facts that never enter the consciousness of average 25 year olds. You are mortal. One day you are going to die. If you do have a life it may not necessarily be of the type you had envisaged in your dreams. You are limited by your own body. And these raised still more questions. How do you come to terms with death? What do you believe happens after you die? Do all things happen for a reason? Is there a reason for this experience? Significantly it taught me that, although surrounded and supported by people, I was alone. This was a tough discovery for an identical twin.

Not only was I shoved towards contemplation of somewhat bigger issues than what to do the next weekend, I also had to look backwards, over my life. With Andrew's help I began to talk about all the experiences that had helped to form me as I am today. I was convinced that there was an emotional component to general health. Without embarking on a long and drawn out self-analysis, there was something I felt a compelling need to do. It was a desire I had long since experienced but that the current situation had made increasingly urgent.

My twin sister and I were adopted at birth. Our natural parents, unmarried and in their early twenties, felt that we would have a better chance in life through adoption. My adoptive parents had bravely taken on two tiny babies, Naomi and I, and we were joined three years later by a further adoptive brother, Nick. Adoption itself was not a big issue for me. I can never remember not knowing that I was adopted. We understood that adopted babies were collected by their parents rather than being born to them. After all, we had collected our brother. One dark winter's evening we had driven through an anonymous London suburb and come back with a new carrycot and a sleeping bundle of blankets in the back of the car. Our parents always told us that we were very special to them because they were able to choose us. Our natural parents, they told us, had been nice people but hadn't been able to look after us. My child's mind had accepted this information unquestioningly but as an adolescent I began to ask more. I had a small white cotton baby dress that had been a gift from my natural mother to my adoptive mother for me. I'd always kept this dress. I still have it today. My mother had an 'adoption file' full of the documents and papers she had gathered. The social workers had collated some general information for us about the people to whom we were genetically linked. I memorised the information about their personal details, how old they were, how tall, what their jobs were, their hobbies and interests.

Later, at university, my interest resurged and I began to talk about tracing my natural mother. However, the problem with being a twin is that there are some situations where very personal decisions cannot be made in isolation. I had considered the issues surrounding my initiative, pointed out by my father, a lawyer specialising in adoptions. Would she have wanted to have put that period of her life behind her? Did she have a new family that would be upset and disrupted by my contact? Would we find we had nothing in common or, worse still, dislike each other? I decided that if I never gave her the chance to meet us then I would never know. She could always say no. My sister strongly disagreed. 'You can't just go barging into someone's life like that' she told me. 'What about her new family?' I wanted to go ahead but felt unable to force such a step on my sister, particularly as she had been ill and I did not want to upset her. So for several years I did nothing. My diagnosis had brought it the surface again. There were things I needed to say to my natural mother. If I didn't do it now I might never get the chance. Particularly now when I had begun to really value my life, I wanted her to know that she had made the right decision and that I had had a good life. I didn't want her to be constantly wondering what happened to the two baby girls she had had so long ago and never get the chance to tell her. For my own curiosity's sake I wanted to know who she was as a person, what was she like? I also wondered if there was a history of cancer in the family. I decided I must act, but I had a practical problem. I was on the other side of the world and tracing people, I assumed, would involve a lot of sifting through records and endless fruitless telephone calls. I mentioned my concerns to my mother. 'I'll see what I can do' she promised.

I thought little more of my request for a couple of weeks until my mother rang one evening. 'I've found her,' she told me, to my complete surprise. I hadn't seriously expected a result, particularly so soon. 'How, where, what happened?' I fired a round of questions off all at once. It had been surprisingly easy, she informed me. She had known that my maternal grandfather was a Methodist vicar. A family friend, another Methodist minister with his own adopted children, had discovered that my grandfather had died some years ago but after contacting the parish's current minister had found that his widow still lived in the area. My maternal grandmother suggested that my adoptive mother contact her son, my uncle. Coincidentally my mother and my natural uncle discovered that they had been at university together. Both teachers, they had obviously chatted for a while and she reported him to be very pleasant. He had suggested that I write to him before he contacted my natural mother.

I sat down immediately, pen and paper in hand. I was poised, ready to start, but how did I begin? It was the first time that anyone had asked me to start with a blank page and tell them about me. There was no history and no knowledge, just an empty sheet of paper. What was I to say? It was rather like writing a CV but more comprehensive and extending right back to the beginning. 'And then there was light.' Did he want to know that I'd joined the Brownies aged seven, that I'd persisted for years with excruciatingly awful sounding violin lessons, the full list of my examination grades in chronological order, or what made me laugh, smile and cry? I settled for a widely edited epistle of my memoirs. I explained to him why I wanted to make contact with my natural mother, his sister, put the letter in the post and prayed that he would tell her.

Australia post and the Royal Mail were on my side. The letter sped its way across the world, arriving in Yorkshire four days later. My natural uncle called me immediately. It was a strange experience talking to a complete stranger on the other side of the world who was, however, so closely related to me. He told me about the family. He had two teenage children, my cousins, and my natural mother had had two more, younger children of her own. She and her family lived down in the south of England.

'What else did you want to know about the family?' he asked me.

I didn't know. For so many years I had been burning with

unanswered questions, now I didn't know where to begin. We talked for a while, me beginning to piece together the edge of the jigsaw about my natural mother and her life. Eventually he volunteered, 'I'll ring her tonight and let her know that we've spoken.'

I could hardly believe that I was so close to my goal. I was too excited to sleep much. The following morning the phone rang.

'Hello' I answered.

'Hello, Rachel? This is Elaine here' the voice at the end replied.

'Oh my God. I can't believe it, I can't believe it's you' we both replied.

'You can't believe how long I've waited for this phone call' she told me.

'You can't believe how long I've been thinking about making it' I responded.

I was totally overwhelmed. We talked and talked. I told her all the things I needed to tell her and she told me all the things I believe she had wanted to explain to us for so long. When we were born she had just graduated, that she had no job and no home, and she would have been unable to provide us with the upbringing she would want us to have. The adoption I realised had been a hard decision for her to make. She'd been so pleased when my parents had wanted us.

'It all happened so smoothly' she remembered 'it just seemed to be the right thing.'

She told me all about my half brother, aged ten, and my half sister, aged six. I told her all about me, my sister, our family and our childhood. There seemed to be too much information to share. We needed hours and hours of time. When the phone call finished I excitedly rang my sister. She was no longer hesitant. She wanted to speak to her immediately. What was she like? Where did she live? What did she look like?

'She's absolutely lovely' I told her.

I searched through my photo albums looking for samples of photos that would be representative of my life. My mother went through her collection and put together a collage of our early years. Elaine had obviously had the same idea. A few days later I received her package of photos. I scrutinised her face. Did she look like me? Maybe the bone structure, possibly the shape of her eyes? It was so hard to tell. There was little recognisable similarity between my sister and me and our half siblings who smiled out of the photos. Her husband had suggested that they make a video and send it over to us. He appeared to be wonderfully accepting of the whole situation. In her accompanying letter Elaine offered to come out and visit me if I would like her to. She also offered, if I needed any bone marrow for the possible mooted bone marrow transfusion Naomi had obviously mentioned to her, that she be tested as a potential donor. She was, I thought, as nice as my mother and the social workers had suggested. I felt that the circle had been completed. There had always been myself and Naomi, and of course our very loving adoptive family, but there had always been a missing chapter which had now been written. I felt I had some roots, I had a history. I could begin to answer the medical question beginning 'Do you have a family history of ...'

A couple of weeks later I was at the post office collecting a parcel. Ripping it open in anticipation, I found videotape and an accompanying letter. Warner Brothers would not, Elaine suspected, be bashing her door down in an urgent hurry, but to the best of her abilities they had produced a videotape.

Slotting the videotape into my machine my natural mother suddenly became real to me. I'd waited for so long to see her. As I watched the tears were rolling down my face. I wasn't quite sure why I was crying, my mixed up emotions just needed an outlet. I felt happiness at seeing her and how lovely she was as a person, yet this was tinged with the sadness that this person was actually still a stranger to me and at the circumstances of our meeting as well as the circumstances of our initial parting. I also cried for the completeness. She'd started off nervously, perching on the edge of her seat, but relaxed into the tape, her body unthawing, gestures and expressions revealing her personality and her warmth. There she was, sitting on her sofa, telling me about her life, our birth and the circumstances surrounding it. It was hard to believe that the woman talking to me from the tape had given birth to me nearly 26 years before. It must have been so difficult for her to sit so calmly and reminisce to a lens. She was dredging back painful and difficult memories in an attempt to anticipate our questions, giving us the information that would give a background to our origins. We no longer just existed, there was a whole story surrounding us. She had some old photos of her and our father in Hyde Park, and some more from a trip to the beach, images that made them seem so much more real as people. She'd kept them in case we had ever wanted them. I wondered whether we looked like him. She said we had his smile in the photographs I'd sent. How did it feel to her to see two young women smiling at you with the smile of someone that you hadn't seen for over 20 years, someone connected with less happy times?

The TV screen propelled me forward into part two of the video.

The rest of her family. The kids were a little camera shy but soon warmed to their task. I was introduced to their two huge black dogs and even got introduced to the hamster. Elaine's husband managed to coax his son into speaking to me in French, amazingly fluently and confidently for a ten year old. As I watched Elaine with her family I realised what a good mother she was. No wonder she had felt she would have been unable to give us the right opportunities so many years before. Now she was obviously capably able to give her children many. They seemed a very happy family unit.

My friends were vividly charting my progress and closely inspected the photos and video for visual similarities between us.

'You should send her a video of yourself and Sydney' one of them suggested.

He enlisted the help of another friend, Jeremy, a drama teacher with creative ideas and, critically, the ability to use a video camera. What would I say? Anything too planned would seem contrived. I didn't want to reiterate my lifetime's CV in yet more detail. I wanted to give her an idea of who I was as a person. By the appointed day my mind was still pretty devoid of ideas. Luckily, Jeremy's was not. He enlisted our help in putting settees on his school's hall stage. He was so unobtrusive with the video camera that I almost forgot that he was there while Anne posed me questions such as:

'What is your idea of your ideal night out?'

'Tell me about the loves in your life.'

'What are you going to do when you get better?'

Watching it back gave me a picture of myself that I hadn't seen for a while. I could feel my ideas, hopes and plans coming through the screen at me. A reaffirmation of how I really was. The words were being spoken by my Star Trek image. Completely hairless. What would she make of me? The photos I'd sent had shown a pretty girl smiling at the camera in a variety of exotic holiday destinations. I worried that the children would be disturbed by my appearance. Could they understand cancer, chemotherapy, hair loss, a bald half sister they had never met? I added a note of caution with the tape, maybe watch it without the children first. I didn't want to scare them. I didn't want to worry Elaine by 'looking sick'. The cancer that had engendered our reunion also complicated it.

The physical changes associated with cancer were obviously not unique to me. One of the hospital social workers suggested that I might be interested in a programme called 'Look Good Feel Better'. It was a programme for female cancer patients to help them deal with image changes that may result from the treatment regimes they were under. I was a little apprehensive at first. I had never really bothered much about make up. I'd been lucky enough to not have to need to. However, the face that stared back at me every time I glanced in the mirror was nothing like the one that I was used to. The 'Look Good Feel Better' seminar was held at the hospital. I entered the large seminar room to find a large table laid out with a host of bottles and tubes, pencils and brushes. Thirty women of all ages were seated around the table in front of large rectangular mirrors. Some still had hair but there was a plethora of headscarves interspersed with a couple of hats. It all looked rather serious. I gingerly took my place. I felt rather like a five-year-old at her mother's dressing table. I giggled with my neighbour as I tried, for the first time in my life, to attempt a full make over. The make up artist rushed to my rescue. She restored my eyebrows for me in the form of eye pencil, my cheeks won back some of their colour that the chemo had washed away (I had been avoiding sunshine due to the photosensitivity created by the drugs). I began to recognise and even to like the face that I was decorating. But enough of faces, we were moving on to hats. Hats I was used to. I used them primarily for hiding under. I had a number of big brimmed and floppy hats that had been carefully chosen to balance my need to see where I was going with my desire to be as well hidden as possible. Since my image had changed I found that my whole body language had adapted with it. I would no longer stride confidently along the street, but shuffle along looking at the floor, conscious that people would be looking at me and wondering 'What's wrong with her?' There were a much greater range of hats on offer than I had allowed myself. I played with the samples. Somehow with my new face they didn't look so bad. We moved on.

Hats completed, the next topic of conversation was wigs. I had in fact purchased a wig. Encouraged by my sister I had tried to recreate my original hairstyle. I wasn't convinced. I felt uncomfortable and conspicuous wearing it. Knowing that it was a wig myself I was convinced that everyone else would be able to spot it. It had a fringe, necessary to hide the false hairline, which I detested. It was hot and itchy in the heat of the Australian summer and so became destined to live out the rest of its life in my underwear drawer. The 'wig lady' plumped for me as her model. My bald head was ideal to fit wigs on to. With my washed out chemo face she evidently believed that I was blonde. She presented me with a head full of the most beautiful long blonde curls. In contrast to my usual short, black bob it was quite a shock but, after getting used to my reflection, I thought I didn't really make such a bad blonde after all. I began to enjoy myself; how would I look as a redhead? I hadn't played with my appearance for a long time. Not many people get the chance to change their hairstyle and colour quite so radically. Many cosmetic companies had contributed their products as a gift to the programme participants so I wandered home, with a lessened fascination for the pavement, clutching a goodie bag that could go some way towards helping me feel more normal.

Four months after my diagnosis, the lull in my treatment allowed me to take stock of things. As well as taking its toll on me, my disease was taking its toll on the rest of my family as well as the friends around me. It was particularly difficult for my sister, my twin, to reconcile herself to the fact that she might lose me. Although independent people, there had always been two of us. She could not imagine a situation where there was only one. She was trying hard to be strong for me. While she had stayed with me for the first few weeks in Sydney I had felt her trying to protect me from the doctors, protect me from the painful tests and treatments. She encouraged me to surround myself with the friends she believed would be supportive, disapproving of those she did not think would help me throughout my illness. Yet I could feel underneath how hard it was for her to have to be so strong. In other ways it was difficult for my mother and father who were miles away in England where it was hard for them to understand what was going on. They could offer very little practical help or advice from such a distance. They were upset that they did not know what was going on. I was upset that they couldn't understand what I was experiencing so could not necessarily offer me the support I felt that I needed. My father could talk his worries through with his wife, but my mother, who was alone, would talk to me about how concerned and frightened she was for me. I was unable to deal with her worries on top of my own. My sister was also only able to cope with her own fears. We suggested that our mother talk to an objective counsellor. There is only so much support that families can give each other in such a distressing and involving situation and no one is an objective listener. I was finding the objective support that I got from Andrew invaluable, I hope and believe that my mother found the same with the local cancer counsellor she saw. Practical familial support for me, once Naomi had gone back to Adelaide, came from Nick. He found the time to come to a lot of different hospital appointments with me. He would run errands when I was too tired or ill to go out. He was available for a hug and the constant reassurance that 'you'll be all right'.

One of the most difficult aspects of my illness was seeing the negative impact it was having on the people around me, how upsetting and distressing it was, the extra burdens which it was placing on them. I knew that I was the cause of these effects, but there was absolutely nothing that I could do to change the situation. Although I recognised that it was not my 'fault' that I had cancer, after all I had not asked for it, I still felt an overwhelming guilt over its impact on those around me. It is so traumatic for those close to a cancer patient to see their loved one suffer and yet be totally unable to do anything to help them. Cancer is so frightening because it does engender such feelings of helplessness. At the outset of my illness, when the picture had been very black, I had been discussing the likely progression of my disease with Dr Norton.

'I do not want to have to go through a lot of pain' I told him. 'I don't want my family to have to see me go through such pain. It would be too much for them. If I'm going to die I want you to let me die with some dignity.'

Of course he had to reply that euthanasia was illegal, but to me it seemed too cruel. How can a supposedly civilised society allow its members to die both with physical pain and the emotional anguish of knowing that their last few weeks, months or even years have caused immeasurable pain and unhappiness to those that are closest to them? I can only believe that those who so oppose the idea of an individual's right to choose when to die have never been faced with a situation in which they could cause so many people, as well as themselves, so much pain.

I was also worrying about the day-to-day burdens I was putting on my friends. I felt so ill-equipped to deal with my own situation, how could any of them manage? My cancer had an ability to permeate so many people's lives. I felt that in every relationship I was doing all the taking and none of the giving. It was as if I was a lead monkey on the backs of my friends, clinging on with claws of steel. Once I articulated my fears to one of them. He thought for a while then commented. 'I think it is a privilege for people to be able to give. We don't get many chances in everyday life do we?' He paused. 'I mean, how often do we really do anything for anyone else?' he asked me. I hadn't thought that maybe others were also gaining through this experience. It made it easier to accept all the giving and the help that people were offering me if I thought about it that way. I began to feel privileged myself in seeing the caring side of people's natures that this context engendered.

Not only were my friends in Australia helping me step-by-step through each day of my illness, my English friends were also offering their love and support. Lucy, a friend since university days, flew out from London to be with me when I had my operation. She also recommended a break away from Sydney for a few days. What I really wanted was a holiday from cancer, but that unfortunately was not one of the options, so we settled for a few days up the coast from Brisbane, at Noosa. Seeing an old friend who had known me so long before I was ill was a double-edged sword. I relaxed into my old self a little, the cancer patient label fading into the background as we reminisced. But I looked at Lucy and her ability to get on a plane and travel across the world, her freedom and independence. I envied her. This time last year I had been like that. I compared myself now, all my plans constructed around my health and my treatment. My wings had not been clipped but completely severed. I had not just flown too close to the sun but I had actually touched it. Her arrival emphasised what I had lost.

My wings may have been clipped but the aeroplane served as a good replacement to whisk us off to our holiday destination. Arriving at the airport I was amazed how I was seemingly unable to deal with 'normal' things. I stood by letting Lucy make all the arrangements. My brain seemed to be full of cancer things. I didn't have any spare capacity to deal with the simple things that would have been commonplace to me beforehand. I still didn't know the exact date of my operation but I was determined not to let its looming presence worry me. I was going to have a few days off. Having installed ourselves in our apartment we rushed down for a preliminary checkout of the beach and headed off to the nearest coffee shop. We had a burning need for cakes, coffee and a long awaited catch up chat. Our cake consuming and gossiping did not last long. We were interrupted mid-sentence by my mobile phone, its ringing cutting sharply through the slow and sleepy afternoon's heat. I knew before I answered it that it would not be good news. My operation had been scheduled for the following week, we needed to be back in Sydney three days later. Our holiday was short but sweet.

CHAPTER 5

All the King's horses – surgery

Organising an operation must be an administrative nightmare. There are so many people involved. Arriving at the hospital I was confronted with a long list of people that I needed to see. There were a number of preliminary tests, forms that needed to be completed, questions to be asked and answered. Despite this, there was a lot of waiting around. Determined not to spend the whole weekend before the scheduled Tuesday sitting in hospital worrying about the operation, I begged for permission to leave. My eventual release was critical to ensure attendance at the pre-operation party that had been organised by a group of friends. So I arrived back at the hospital on Monday morning, still full with the food and drink they had prepared to sustain me over the following week and comforted by reassuring stories of painless stays in intensive care and successful operations.

This second hospital was a more recent building than the older style buildings where I had had my initial operation and treatment. The ward had a row of two bedded rooms and was light and airy. Lucy had equipped me with her portable CD player and a mountain of supermarket snacks to save me from the hospital food. We turned my bed into a card table and covered it in biscuit crumbs. We made ourselves quite at home. Our games were interrupted by the appearance of a variety of white-coated doctors. The first to arrive was the registrar to the neurosurgeon. Until that point I had not appreciated that there would be two teams working on my head simultaneously. I had met the ENT surgeon, Dr Jarman, who would be operating, at the head and neck clinics. I also knew that Dr Haxell would be present. He had been invited by his colleague, Dr Jarman, and kindly accepted. It was reassuring to know that there would be someone there who knew me as a person rather than a body on the table. I felt much safer. But this was the first time I had heard talk of a neurosurgeon.

The registrar informed me that I was to have what they termed a cranio-facial resection. He explained carefully the part of the procedure that he would be involved with. They would cut across the top of my head, almost ear to ear. They would then peel my skin forward and drill into the section of bone in my forehead. They would then remove this circle of bone completely, enabling them to lift up my brain and provide the required access for Dr Jarman. I was stunned. This did not sound like the kind of operation that would leave me with 'a small scar down the side of my nose'. The neurosurgeon would be along later, he told me. I could direct any further questions to him, but he warned me that he 'shoots from the hip'. I prepared myself for a monster. Dr Ellington, it turned out, was not a monster at all. He was a very smartly dressed and efficiently kind Chinese man. He went through the general surgical procedure again in further detail. He then began to explain the risks. There was a risk that the spinal fluid could begin to leak as a result of the surgery. There was of course a risk of infection and potentially meningitis. Removal of the bone may leave dents in my forehead. I may experience agitation and personality disturbances and of course there was a risk of epilepsy. I tried to digest this list. 'Anything else?' I queried, fervently hoping not. That apparently was it. These were not high risks but he had to tell me that there was a chance that these eventualities could occur. He smiled at me, 'See you tomorrow' and quietly disappeared. I was rather shaken.

'It's OK' Lucy reassured me. 'Those things won't happen to you.'

I hoped not.

A little while later another registrar appeared. Dr Dawson was a softly spoken and gentle mannered South African. His job was to complete the rest of the surgical jigsaw puzzle, explaining the remainder of the procedure. He began carefully and slowly, demonstrating on his own face. They would cut down the right hand side of my nose, from the corner of my eye to the bottom of my nostril. They would fracture my nose towards the left of my face. This would give them side on access, as well as the entry point created by the neurosurgical team through my forehead. They would then remove the tumour and surrounding tissue before reconstructing my head. They would take some tissue from my outer thigh in order to do this. It sounded like a nursery rhyme, with me starring as Humpty Dumpty being 'put back together again' by this team of clinically garbed men. The operation was far more major than I had realised. I would be in intensive care for a number of days. If I did experience significant pain I was assured that I would not remember it. I was unsettled by the idea of losing a week of my life through a drug induced haze.

'What about my neck?' I asked Dr Dawson.

He looked at me rather blankly.

'I have tumours in the lymph nodes in my neck' I continued. 'I was expecting them to be taken out as well, at least I thought so...' I trailed off as he continued to look at me blankly. 'It doesn't say anything about that on these forms' he puzzled. 'I'll check that for you.'

The impact of what the surgery really meant in practical terms had hit me hard. I had made a decision about notional surgery at a future date. I had reached that date and now I was being confronted by the gruesome details. Is it really necessary? Do I really need to go through this? Some of the doctors in the head and neck clinic had believed that radiotherapy alone would be sufficient, maybe they were right? I began to panic. I needed to know why surgery was the better option, why the eventual decision had been to recommend a combination of treatment. I thought over all he had told me. I was overwhelmed by all the details. For my own peace of mind I knew that I had to believe that this was absolutely necessary before I put myself through it. I asked if I could possibly see my radiotherapist, Dr Newbury. Yes, that was possible, they would arrange for me to go down. A few moments later a porter appeared with a wheelchair.

'What's that for?' I asked.

'For you to go down to radiotherapy in' I was told.

I was offended. I didn't need a wheelchair. I couldn't care less about their arguments for hospital regulations and such like, I had legs and I was using them.

Dr Newbury was wonderful. Uncharacteristically patient, he produced a skull and showed me exactly what they were going to do; he explained far more comprehensively the reasons why he believed that surgery was necessary to give me the optimal chance of survival. I asked him whether the lymph nodes would also need to be removed. Most definitely, he replied and he assured me that he would establish this with the medical team.

'You'll be all right' he reassured me, patting my hand. 'A few days in intensive care, and then you'll be back on the ward. You'll probably be out of here in less than two weeks.'

I took myself back up to the ward to find Geraldine, Sarah's mother, sitting beside my bed. I was so pleased to see her.

'I've come to make sure you're all right' she told me.

She'd arrived at just the right time. Within minutes we were whisked away down to the intensive care unit. Patients and their relatives were toured around the unit in order to familiarise them with the environment. I could understand why. It was very different to the ordinary ward. There were many more screens and monitors, respirators, drips, tubes, and all the things that TV hospital dramas show. It was very different off-screen. It was so quiet. I was pleased that Geraldine was with me. This was all quite normal to her, she was able to embellish on our tour guide's explanations. I watched the still and silent bodies, encased in their white sheets, gently rising and falling to the beat of their respirator. In a couple of days that would be me, a shrouded sculpture. I could not imagine it. I felt cold. I was glad to leave. Back on the ward I timidly began to ask Geraldine some questions.

'Will I be on a respirator?'

'What will it be like having a tracheotomy?'

'How will they know if I'm in pain?'

'Will I remember anything?'

'How long will I have to be there?'

Somehow it was easier to ask someone I liked and trusted. Geraldine inspired in me a feeling of confidence in her capability as a nurse. She stayed with me for a while until the anaesthetist arrived.

'Would you please leave?' he asked her abruptly.

We looked at each other.

'I'm here instead of her family' Geraldine began to explain. He ushered her out. I was appalled. He hadn't asked me whether I wanted anyone to stay with me.

'Well, she didn't want to go' he started conspiratorially.

'No' I replied, 'but she is a friend and a nurse, I feel comfortable with her here.'

I appreciated that he was probably busy but that did not excuse his rudeness. His manner suggested that he felt a real power differential between himself and his patients and their friends and relatives. Once he got talking he really wasn't too bad, he managed to explain his role in the following day's events, fired off a few questions and gave me a quick examination. I was relieved when he had gone and Geraldine, now accompanied by Sarah, was permitted back in.

By now I had a pretty clear idea of what the following day would involve. I had met the surgeons and the anaesthetist, I had seen the intensive care unit which would be my abode for the subsequent days. Everything I needed to know had been explained to me. Now I was scared. I felt as if I had jumped out of a plane without a parachute and was falling in slow motion just waiting to hit the ground, knowing that it would hurt like hell. Our picnic dinner, on our makeshift picnic bed-table, was a symbolic Last Supper to me.

We talked about other things, avoiding all mention of the coming events. Dr Dawson reappeared. More administration was required. The amount of paper surrounding a hospital admission and associated surgery is astounding, but also reassuring. I was glad to know they had the important detail duplicated on so many different forms, at least someone might notice. This time Dr Dawson needed my consent. He had to check that I had a full understanding of the cranio-facial resection and neck dissection that would be carried out the following day. He told me that the doctors who would be present would be the neurosurgical team I had already met – Dr Ellington and his assistant. Dr Dawson may be that assistant or it could be 'a guy who is over from The States'. Dr Dawson looked tired. Sarah asked him if he'd had an early start that morning. He replied that he had not been to bed the night before, and looked set to have another very late night. I turned to look at him and said, semi-joking, 'You're not operating on me tomorrow then'. It does seem that there is something wrong with our sense of proportion when we expect our young doctors to work such incredible hours (and that is coming from a management consultant) and then competently and capably spend the whole following day deconstructing somebody's head and then reconstructing it again in the correct order. I had no doubt that Dr Dawson was very competent and committed but all humans have their limitations as regards fatigue, and I have only one head.

By the time the paperwork had been completed I was exhausted myself. Not physically exhausted but my mental capacity had been severely stretched. There had been so much to take in, and a considerable proportion of my brain had been purely dedicated to worrying about the following day. I burst into tears.

'I didn't know that it was going to be like this. I really don't want to have this, I'm scared' I wailed to Sarah, Lucy and Dr Dawson.

I knew I was behaving like a child, illustrating perfectly the phrase 'tired and emotional'. Sarah fished out a tissue.

'This time tomorrow it will be all over' she comforted.

All over, but I would be in intensive care, drugged out of my brain with a tracheotomy in my throat. I was scared of that too. I carried on wailing. I just needed to get everything out of my system. Dr Dawson got me some sleeping pills and I trundled off down the corridor to my bed. Sarah and Lucy sat talking gently to me until I fell asleep, drifting away hazily as the drugs began to work their magic. The girls promised to be back the next morning at 5.30 am, before I went down to theatre.

I awoke from a deep, deep nothingness to see a small, furry face with blue eyes snuzzling up to my face. A little pink tongue protruded and licked my nose. It smelt of cat food. 'Molly', I exclaimed as my favourite little creature scrambled into my bed and burrowed down next to me, happy to find a familiar smell. Sarah had smuggled Molly into the hospital for me. She'd bundled her into a basket and hidden her under some clothing, only stopping to show one of the nurses who'd been in on the act. Molly, sensibly scared by all the strange hospital smells and noises and an unfamiliar car ride, had laid low and was relieved to find her 'mum' at the other end. We had a nice twenty-minute doze together until they came to give me my premed, and the rather unattractive surgical socks that were my uniform. A small injection and a minute later Molly, along with the girls and the rest of the world, vanished out of my sight.

Apparently, I had been awake as I was wheeled down to the operating theatre. Dr Haxell had appeared and comfortingly held my hand, talking to me until I went under, but that is all lost to me now. The last thing I remembered was being curled up in bed with little Molly.

I woke up, and my feet hurt. They were aching as if I had just completed a fifty-mile hike, all uphill. I tried to tell someone about my feet but I couldn't speak. I slipped back out of consciousness. I had anticipated losing all recollection of the events which took place while I was in intensive care. Surprisingly, I can remember quite a lot about these days, and Geraldine and Naomi have been able to fill me in on a lot of what was missing. It was a very strange puzzle to piece together. Another very early recollection was reaching up to touch my neck. I felt the right hand side with my right hand. Perfect. There were no dressings or bandages. My neck was untouched, pure, smooth skin. I must have been very distressed by this discovery. I touched my neck many times, checking. I remember Dr Ellington, Dr Dawson and Dr Newbury all appearing at times during the following days to explain to me why they had not removed the lymph nodes. I remember their faces, and long and earnest explanations, designed to reassure me, but I can't for the life of me remember anything they actually said to me.

Communication for me took the form of a magic board. I could scribble my piece on to the board and then wave it around frantically to attract the attention of someone to read it. Apparently I did a lot of scribbling. Geraldine told me that I had been very distressed the evening after the surgery. They had not expected me to be conscious, let alone so alert and anxious. I may well have been experiencing some agitation as a result of the surgery, but the situation was painful and scary, which would explain my anxiety equally well. My chief fear was related to the tracheotomy and the respirator. It felt so strange to be breathing through a tube in my neck. I was terrified that if I went to sleep I would stop breathing. Geraldine patiently held my hand and explained that I didn't need to worry, that I wouldn't stop breathing, and, even if I did, the respirator would breathe for me. I don't think I was convinced. They pumped more and more sedatives into my body, but it was a long while until I would give in to them and go back to sleep.

I hated that tracheotomy. With horrible regularity a suction tube would be inserted down into my lungs to remove any mucus. It was an uncomfortable experience and I would count the seconds until it was over. I also found it difficult to breathe. On one occasion when I got upset, I found that my chest was constricting and I just couldn't get enough air in. I panicked, making it worse. I was sure it was an asthma attack. The nurse tried to convince me, rightly, that it wasn't but I couldn't calm down. Being unable to breathe was one of the worst experiences I had in intensive care. Having the trachy even stopped me from being able to cry properly. The doctor was called to check and reassure me that it really wasn't asthma. The whole episode made me so exhausted that I clung to the nurse. It was a relief when I found sanctuary in drifting back off to sleep.

At one point, I remember being told that I was going to have a CT scan. A week or so later, back on the ward, I asked when I was to have it. They laughingly replied that I had already had it, I had obviously been oblivious to the whole thing. I had missed out on an amusing situation, Geraldine told me. For some reason I was scared of having the scan and wanted Geraldine to come with me. The problem was that I would not let go of her hand. They had quite a debacle trying to squeeze me, on a trolley, hooked up to my entourage of machines and dragging Geraldine, who is quite substantial, beside me, all out together through the door. It must have been quite a manoeuvre, I was sorry to have been present in body but absent in mind.

It could understandably be worse for many of the relatives and friends of patients who are in ICU than it is for the patients themselves. I was so drugged that I did lose, thankfully, a lot of the experience in a blur. Apparently I had a lot of visitors, but many of them vanished into my haze. One friend said that the whole experience was so upsetting that she couldn't come to see me again. Geraldine was fantastic. She stayed with me for a long time that first night. I had, they told me, got very distressed every time she tried to go. I must have trusted her and felt safe with her to protect me from this painful and strange environment which I had woken up to. My flatmates reported that I had seemed quite alert and like myself. They had been laughing and joking with me about the doctors, and I had happily responded via my magic board. I can't even remember seeing them. However, my sister found it very difficult seeing me in pain. She spent a lot of time trying to help me communicate but did on occasion act as a censor to my magic board. I had angrily written 'Get that bloody nurse out of here', I can't remember what that 'bloody nurse' had actually done now, but my scribblings were duly wiped away until I rephrased myself more acceptably. Dr Haxell's wife, Gill, came to visit me several times. She tried to protect me from the stream of visitors I seemed to be receiving. She tried very hard not to mind the medical procedures she was witnessing but as the nurses began to remove some sort of tube or drain she murmured 'I'm beginning to feel a little faint.' I scribble on my magic board 'I don't think Gill will want to see this.' The nurse suggested a seat outside. That was the first time that I became aware how difficult it was for other people to have to look on as things were being done to me. I have to admire the strength that Sarah, Naomi and Lucy had, coming back to see me time and time again.

I did have one surprise visitor who managed to amuse Geraldine. Weeks earlier my Scottish friend Ralph had had a Burns night supper. We had all duly dressed in tartan, eaten haggis, consumed too much whisky, danced reels and read poetry. One of the other guests had been a doctor. We hadn't spoken much that night but she had heard that I was in hospital and suddenly appeared in my room.

'Hello Rachel. How are you?'

I opened my one eye that was functioning, the other was swollen closed. I peered at her, feeling my lack of contact lenses. She went on talking for a while.

'Who are you?' I had eventually asked, via my board, feeling that I should recognise her but in fact totally devoid of any recollection of knowing her. Geraldine found that priceless as Abigail reminded me of when we had met.

'She said she wanted to go for a drink with you sometime!' Geraldine reminded me later. Make a mental note, I said to myself, next time you go in to intensive care remember to take your diary.

I never really got to grips with the machines that had temporarily become part of me. I don't recall many of them being disconnected but over a few days I was gradually released from my chains. The one that caused me the most anxiety was the machine which controlled the analgesic. It kept going off sporadically, rather like an alarm clock, its beeps panicking me until the nurse came to sort things out. What I didn't realise for a long while was that these beeps were just routine and did not mean, as I imagined, that something had gone horribly wrong. I would lie, body rigid, waiting for something awful to happen, before the nurses, at their leisure, came to silence it again.

I don't recall the trip from the intensive care unit back to the ward. I do still have vivid recollections of being very, very sick. The doctors were worrying that it was meningitis, but I think it was actually just a reaction to the morphine. Even through the drugs I was really miserable. It was equally bad for my sister who had to leave me in the middle of my sickness to return to her job in Adelaide, left with her final picture of me in such a state. My memories of those couple of days consist of waking up, being horribly sick and then drifting back into an exhausted sleep, only to be woken up by another bout of sickness. I remember the doctors gently trying to coax me to drink something. I tried to sip at apple juice, and cautiously at some milk. It all came back up. 'What can I eat?' I scrawled miserably on my magic board. I didn't seem to be able to take anything. Being sick with a tube stuck through your throat is not a comfortable business. I was as relieved as they were when I was switched to pethidine, the vomiting ceased and I was able to begin to stomach water.

I was vaguely aware of my visitors. I would scribble notes to them, and then fall asleep during their replies, waking up to find them gone again. I had lost all sense of timing, not knowing how long I had been like this. The days, along with the dreaded nights, merged into one another. The nights felt very long and stifling. I hated the darkness broken by the noise of hospital activities and the endless beeping of the machines. At least there were people around me during the days. Their presence comforted me, helping to take the edge off my anxiety and pain. I wondered if they realised how much I needed their visits. Sometimes there were too many people and I felt exhausted by the constant need to be conscious, to concentrate and try to make some sense of what they were saying. I knew that I would rather be tired by these people, my friends, than to be without them.

It was several more days until I realised how shocking their visits must have been for them. A couple of friends told me later that they had been unable to find me. Walking through the ward, checking every room, they had drawn a blank. Eventually, tracking down a nurse they had been directed back to one of the rooms they had passed, to find an unrecognisable body sleeping in a bed. Another friend had actually fainted. The nurses had already despatched a wheelchair to take her to casualty before she had gathered herself together enough to assure them that this really wasn't necessary. The first time I got out of bed and to the shower room I understood why. I stared at the bruised and swollen face with which the mirror confronted me. 'Oh my God, is that me?' I had had no image in my mind's eye of how this operation would have affected my face. I was totally unrecognisable. How could that grotesquely bruised and swollen face belong to me? I looked like Frankenstein, metal clips across my head, stitches down the side of my nose. The skin surrounding my eye was a deep plum colour. It wasn't my face. It was some sort of gargoyle, hardly a face at all. I didn't want to look at it. For the rest of my stay I tried to avoid mirrors.

Gradually, the various drips, drains and lines which were hooked into various parts of my body were removed. It was a great relief when my tracheotomy was removed and my powers of speech were restored to me. Although I had to hold my fingers over the gaping hole that remained, I was able to communicate properly again. I no longer had to undertake the stilted conversation using the magic board, but could respond with my own voice. I tried my first croak and was surprised to find out that it worked, I could still speak. I grinned at the doctors. I have never liked the sound of my own voice so much. As I was unhooked, I was able to be more mobile. I could move around in bed without tying myself up in knots, I could even get up and walk down to the bathroom.

My first shower was rather like a car wash. Having been unwashed for over a week, I felt groggy to the core. I begged for a shower. The nurses were short on time but a couple of visiting friends offered their services. I was still attached to the patient controlled analgesic machine. These machines far outdo the supermarket trolley for bad steering. However, it served perfectly adequately as a crutch to lean on. I hobbled down the corridor to the shower room. I sat naked in a chair and trying to avoid soaking my mechanical appendage, I covered myself in soap with my free hand. Anne then hosed me down with the shower. It felt good, as if the water was cleansing my whole body, washing out the tension as well as just my skin. I struggled out of the hospital gown that had made me look like a prisoner, and into a nightie of my own. I was transformed, instantaneously more human but exhausted by our ten minute adventure. I zig zagged myself and my machine back to bed.

The one common and enduring complaint about hospitals is the food. This hospital was no exception. Mercifully, I had avoided their cuisine for a week. Lack of consciousness and extreme sickness had

had its advantages. Now I had to begin to eat. My friends, taking a quick look at what was supposed to help regain my strength, took pity. I received regular food parcels from their mothers, designed to tempt me into hunger. My brother on the other hand was far less fussy. The hospital meals continued to arrive, as did my brother with perfect timing. He couldn't afford to be picky, he pointed out to Sarah and I between mouthfuls one evening, as we sat watching him in astonishment as he inhaled a tray of food with gusto. He was, after all, travelling on a budget. We shook our heads and pulled questioning faces at each other as he happily carried on chewing.

My days were considerably brightened by a dear American friend, Nancy, arriving back in Australia. After flying up to Sydney, she arrived at the hospital with bags of food, piles of magazines and her wonderful smile. She was a breath of fresh air to me. We just 'hung out' and chatted, not necessarily about cancer but about new ideas, life changes and pure gossip. It was good to see her. I found it interesting to see the different ways in which people handled me in hospital, how they reacted to illness and the whole environment. Some friends felt that I would rather not see them, that they would be disturbing me if they visited and would get in the way. Others were determined to do whatever they could, visiting me often, bringing in gifts of food and flowers, anything that might make my situation more pleasant and comfortable. It must have been incredibly difficult for any of them to know the 'right' way to react. I know that I needed people with me, but others who have experienced similar situations have wanted to be left well alone. I felt that the support I got from my friends was vital to my recovery. One older nurse, objecting to my constant stream of visitors, complained that they might be disturbing the lady in the adjacent bed.

'You don't know what she's going through' she admonished me.

True, I thought to myself, upset. But this nurse obviously had absolutely no idea what I was going through. I was 25 years old, overseas, away from my family, coping with a major operation and a life-threatening disease. She had no concept of the fact that my constant stream of visitors was what was keeping me from falling apart. Although I did feel desperately sorry for the lady in the adjacent bed, my sympathies were somewhat lessened by the fact that she was a heavy smoker, and would be out on the balcony smoking at any opportunity, despite the fact that she had throat cancer. Some people choose to go through this, I thought. They know that an experience like this is a possibility yet they still go on smoking. It must be so frustrating for doctors treating their disease. Where is the motivation to help people who do not want to help themselves? This lady had a rasping voice and an awful rattling, chesty cough that I would listen to all night. She had certainly damaged her body through the years of her habit. I made all my smoking friends who visited listen to her cough; it was enough to make at least two of them quit.

My stay in hospital made me realise how outdated my view of nurses was. I had anticipated nurses as rather comforting figures who would relate to their patients as people, rather than bodies in beds. There was one very maternal sort of nurse on the ward, and a couple of Irish girls who were both really warm and friendly. They were always comforting to be around. But to others I could have been a wax model and I don't think they would have realised the difference. Generally, nursing seemed to be far more of a technical occupation than I had imagined. Of course, with nursing degrees becoming the norm and medical technology increasing, it is hardly surprising that the job of the nurse is rapidly changing. All the nurses I came across, without exception, were highly competent but desperately busy. These developments no doubt benefit the patient in terms of the technical treatment that they receive but I wondered if maybe some of the more traditional caring aspects were being forced out by time constraints.

After I had been back on the ward for a few days, Dr Dawson appeared and suggested that I get up and take some exercise.

'After all' he pointed out, 'even I'd be ill if I lay in bed for two weeks and there's nothing wrong with me.'

So I got up. Swinging my legs round on to the floor, I tested my balance and prepared myself to begin. I happily trundled up and down the corridor a couple of times, trying out my 'bad' leg, the one from which they had taken the muscle covering for the reconstructive work on my head. Fortunately, it seemed to be holding up all right. After retracing my steps a number of times I began to feel trapped, caged like an animal, as if the walls of the hospital were closing in on me. Was the outside world still there? I had only been away from it for a few days but I was beginning to feel cut off from the hustle and bustle of its everyday normality. I decided to try the balcony, hoping to catch a reassuring glimpse of the world going about its business as usual. I walked slowly up and down, savouring the lungfuls of fresh air, looking all around me, valuing the distances, enjoying the space between me and the sky. At the end of the balcony I spotted some stairs. Stair climbing, now that would be good exercise, I thought, thinking about step classes and the stair machines in gyms, that'd get my muscles moving again. How far up should I go, six floors, maybe eight? I began climbing six or eight floors – forget it, I couldn't even manage six to eight steps. The leg muscle which had been operated on was throbbing with pain. I hoped going down wouldn't be so bad. It was. I clung to the banister hopping on my good leg.

I hadn't been able to make the mental adjustments I needed to deal with the effects of my surgery. If someone said exercise to me that usually meant go for a run, go and get out of breath and sweat a bit. So I had just watered that down a bit, but obviously not sufficiently. I talked about this with Andrew later. I wanted to be able to enjoy living an active life again. Doing exercise daily was an established part of my routine. For the first time in my life my body wouldn't let me. It had been through too much, so many drugs, so much surgery. It simply couldn't do what I wanted it to do.

'You need to reframe your exercise' he advised. 'Keep exercise as part of your routine but make it manageable. You don't have to go for a run. At the moment, walking up the stairs is probably the same for you as running used to be.' He continued, pointing out 'you need to exercise for different reasons, not for aerobic fitness but to feel your muscles stretch and because you enjoy being outside in the fresh air.'

He was right, but it was difficult to do. It was probably as hard for me to lose my coping mechanism, exercising, as it was for the lady in the next door bed to me to give up her coping mechanism of smoking, even though it was killing her.

So the days passed and I whiled away my final days on the ward, reading, talking to friends and walking up and down the balcony, trying to build up some stamina. I was amazed how much my leg muscles had wasted by a mere ten days in bed. I had received many, many beautiful flowers. I sat surrounded by them.

'Don't they smell lovely?' one of the doctors commented to me.

'I don't know. I can't smell' I replied.

The operation had robbed me of my sense of smell. He looked awkward.

'Still, they are pretty, aren't they?' I agreed.

The mural of their colours made an enriching contrast to the stark empty white of the hospital room walls. It was as if I was sitting in a tabernacle of flowers, engulfed in the good wishes of my friends, from Australia and England, and work colleagues, from the offices in both countries. Some of my colleagues, committed Christians, were regularly, they informed me, holding weekly prayer sessions for me at work on Friday mornings. Regardless of my own religious views I found it both touching and comforting to know that their thoughts were with me.

At the beginning of my illness, two of these colleagues had asked if they could come round and pray with me. Although their religious beliefs are not necessarily in line with my own, I happily invited them over and was pleased to see them again. They prayed for some time, beginning in English, and then lapsing into 'speaking in tongues', which sounded to me something like a cross between Hebrew and Romanian. They laid their hands over where my tumour was as they prayed to God to make it disappear. I was moved by the strength of their faith and myself strengthened to know that they wished so hard for my recovery. I was a little uneasy about their speaking in tongues. I was not sure why it happened and what its significance was, but whatever they were saying it was a way for them to express how they were feeling. It was the sentiment that mattered.

Before I left the hospital I needed to have my stitches removed. First the ones in my nose, then the ones in my leg. After that they turned their attention to my head. Just as one of the nurses was about to begin unclipping the staples, my friend Diane arrived.

'Hi Di' I greeted her. 'I'm really glad you're here. Now you can distract me as they pull the clips out.'

I pulled up a chair for her. The nurse reappeared with her staple removers and turned me around on the bed, giving her easy access to my head. Fortunately she did a pretty good job, it was a relatively painless process. I chatted away to Di as the nurse worked away, until I realised I was getting no response, Di was no longer there. As soon as the nurse had removed the last clip I went to find her. She was on the chair outside my room looking green and pale. 'Are you all right?' I asked her, worried by her rather dubious colouring.

'I just couldn't watch, it looked awful' she apologised. 'Didn't it hurt?'

'Hardly felt a thing' I replied.

She wasn't convinced. I was so relieved to have her company I hadn't thought how watching the performance would be for her. I'll have to bear that in mind, I thought, hoping there wouldn't be a next time.

I was duly fixed up with my medication and follow-up appointments and discharged. What a relief to be able to go back home. My friend Anne had decreed that she was coming to stay for the weekend.

'I'm not leaving you on your own' she told me, arriving with armfuls of newspapers and groceries.

'I'll be fine' I had assured her.

Secretly I was very pleased to see her. It felt strange to have my liberty again. The nights with uninterrupted sleep were blissful. I have no idea how anyone ever sleeps in hospitals. There are constant crashes, bangs and callings, not to mention the sporadic beeps of machines, bursting through the darkness like bouts of machine gun fire. I took sleeping pills every night I was there just to get a few hours rest. I loved the luxury and indulgence of my own bed and the comparative quiet. It was good to be home.

I was very conscious of going out of the house. My face was still so bruised and swollen, and the scar across my head was very unsightly. At least that could be covered by a hat. I spent a lot of time reading books and watching videos. But try as I might I couldn't stay in for the next year or two waiting for the scars to fade. I was shy of people I didn't know very well coming to visit. My illness was now, quite literally, engraved on my face. Only doctor's appointments forced me out of the house. My trachy was not healing well. Sarah suggested going to see her GP to see what he could do about it.

'He's very funny' she told me, and he was.

I wasn't sure if it was what he said, or just how he was, but we both left his surgery giggling. Spotting my brother, who had accompanied us and who for economic purposes (not having to purchase shampoo) had shaved his head, the doctor gravely asked us if it was genetic.

I also had follow-up appointments to see my surgeons. Nick was insistent that he should drive me up to Dr Jarman's consulting rooms. I was adamant that I could go by myself but Nick was determined to accompany me. Dr Jarman was very pleased with his handiwork and beamed at me across the desk. I believe he had every reason to be so proud, Dr Haxell had apparently returned from the operation singing his praises, amazed at what an art form his surgery had been. I was also very appreciative of his skills. The nurses had also rated him. 'If I was going to let anyone open up my head it'd be him' one of them had assured me. He quickly checked me over. All fine.

'You're not driving yet?' he asked me.

I looked at him blankly.

'Well no', I replied, 'but...' I had been thinking about it, it hadn't occurred to me that I shouldn't.

'You should be all right to drive in a couple of weeks if you haven't experienced any epileptic fits. You haven't had any so far?'

'No'

I was relieved that I hadn't driven. No one had suggested to me that I shouldn't up until then. He moved on to discuss the operation and began to draw me pictures, to clarify exactly what he had done. It really helped for me to be able to visualise exactly what had happened. I needed to realise what had been done to understand my current condition. Dr Haxell helped me further when, inviting me round for dinner one night, he showed me a surgical textbook with photographs of a cranio-facial resection. I had looked at the pictures in an almost detached but interested way. Although I knew that this had happened to me, I couldn't quite relate the photographs to the inside of my own head.

I was worried about the epileptic fits.

'How will I know if I've had one?' I'd asked Dr Jarman.

'Well, you won't' he told me, 'but the people around you will.'

I wondered what I could do to avoid them. Dr Jarman had prescribed me some anti-epilepsy drugs but these were not having a good effect. They made me feel very drugged and I would often fall into a deep, deep sleep in the middle of the day, finding it impossible to fight my way back out into wakefulness. Thankfully he allowed me to stop them. The answer came from a Chinese herbalist, who was not in fact Chinese at all. By the sound of his faint accent I guessed that he may have been South African. He was a short, rounded man whose office was a bit of an anomaly – traditional, heavy wooden furniture with delicate Chinese decorations. He worked closely with a Tokyo-based doctor and had developed, he said, herbal remedies to act against tumour cells and also against epilepsy. He, like the acupuncturist, conducted his diagnosis by wrist pulses and examination of the tongue. I had nothing to lose by taking his rather bitter tasting herbs. I certainly had more energy from the Ginseng they contained and whether by luck or for any other reason, I never had an epileptic fit.

My follow-up appointment with Dr Ellington was miles away in an area of Sydney which I had never visited. A friend's parents, both in the middle of writing books, so with reasonably flexible schedules, kindly agreed to drive me there. We travelled out on a major highway through the suburbs, past car sales rooms and endless single storied homes. The suburbs of Sydney sprawl for miles.

'This is where Shane comes for his holidays' Marg cheerfully informed me.

I looked around me. Who on earth would want to come here for their holidays? I made polite noises, wondering who Shane was and what was wrong with him; they must have some very peculiar friends. Then, as Kev spoke, I glanced towards a building on my left, the RSPCA dogs kennels.

'Shane is our dog' he told me.

Ahhah. The penny dropped.

We waited at the surgery for a long time. Eventually my name was called. I was in and out of the consulting room in less than eight minutes. I emerged rather shell-shocked.

'What did he say?' they asked me.

'I have to have another operation.'

I had not expected anything like this. I had just got over the last one, I didn't want to go through it all again. To me the word operation was synonymous with major surgery with days in intensive care. Dr Ellington had had a quick look up my nose, 'just a small operation' he'd assured me. I did not regard any operation as small.

I also had a growing concern which itself was gnawing at me like a tumour. It was about the lymph nodes in my neck. I had expected them to be removed and was increasingly disconcerted that they hadn't been. Something wasn't right. I just had a gut feeling that they should have come out. After all Dr Newbury had explained why they should be removed before my first operation but I didn't see what had changed. I had asked Dr Ellington why the nodes had not been removed but I couldn't remember what he had told me when I was in intensive care. He explained that tumour in soft tissue was different to the tumour at the primary site, as regarded treatment. Irradiation would be fine, he assured me. I wasn't convinced, the literature that I had read suggested otherwise. I queried his assurance. No, really, radiotherapy would be fine. I worried all the way home about it.

'The worst thing about this is the anxiety' Marg mused.

I decided to call Dr Norton. I had not spoken to him for a while but I hoped that maybe he could give me an objective view.

'Soft tissue is not different' he told me, 'not in the case of your disease because it is such an aggressive tumour.'

I knew that he was right. I felt so confused. It was as if it was happening all over again. Nobody agreed with each other and I didn't know what I should do. I desperately wanted someone to take the lymph nodes out but I didn't know how to go about it. I worried and fretted all that night. Early the following morning I called Dr Newbury. I told him what Dr Ellington had told me and how Dr Norton disagreed.

'What you told me the day before the operation' I asked him. 'Why has that changed? Why wouldn't you take my lymph nodes out now?'

Dr Newbury was irate. Maybe I had got him at a bad time. He began a rather vague and waffly explanation and then he lost his temper with me.

'Look Rachel, I really don't know. I haven't spoken to Dr Ellington yet. Come in and see me tomorrow.'

The phone call ended.

Later that afternoon Nancy came round for a visit.

'How are you? she asked, unleashing from me a flood of tears, directly into the tea I was making her.

'I just don't know what to do.' I sobbed, letting out all my frustration and confusion. 'I keep getting different answers and I don't know who is right, I don't know what to do.'

Nancy hugged me as I cried, on and on. I was still feeling low from my first operation. I didn't feel able to make decisions and push for information. I just wanted someone to pick me up and help me, to sort everything out.

'Right,' she said as, having soaked the front of her shirt, I showed signs of stopping sniffing, 'have you got a pen and paper?'

She made several lists of the questions that I needed to ask each of the doctors I was seeing. Nancy was a banker at that time and I could see her business training coming out in her methodical approach. It was the approach that I would use towards my clients. Why couldn't I do this for myself? Somehow it was too personal, I could not be objective and I felt increasingly overwhelmed. I needed someone to help me.

I don't think the next day was a much better one as far as Dr Newbury was concerned. He was obviously very busy. He rushed into the room and told me that they were going to operate, they had agreed at last. He had to rush off to a meeting.

'Never mind' I told him, 'I'll wait, I've got plenty of time and I need to understand this.'

I had Nancy's list of questions burning a hole in my pocket. I needed answers to them and I wasn't going to be dismissed back home to worry and fret. He humphed and disappeared.

I was left with Caroline, the oncology sister. We chatted for a while. She remembered our previous meetings and asked after my brother and sister. Her brother, my age, had cancer. She had some idea what I was going through. Caroline was an ideal support to Dr Newbury. Her calmness and polished people skills enabled her to fill a need for patients that was not Dr Newbury's forte.

'Make sure you ask him everything you want to,' she counselled. 'He's difficult to pin down so you have to get him to give you the time you need.'

Five minutes later he was back.

'Meeting's off' he announced airily.

He sat down. I began to ask him my questions. Once seated he was able to give me the explanation that I was seeking. He had always believed that they should remove the lymph nodes, he still believed that he could feel them. The surgeons could not feel them. They laughingly referred to the condition of 'Newbury-nodes', which were actually imaginary. The initial surgery had gone on longer than expected so the surgeons had made the decision not to remove them. I guess this had put Dr Newbury in a difficult position having only the previous afternoon given me a very eloquent explanation as to why they should be removed. He supported Dr Ellington in confirming that soft tissue would be different in most head and neck cancers but that this was not a head and neck cancer. So the argument was settled, I was to have my nodes removed. They would perform a neck dissection. So I finally had the information I needed. I was glad that I had been on a training course on handling difficult clients as I had consciously been bringing those techniques into play to get my answer.

So just when I was beginning to feel better and up to doing things again I was back in hospital. Cancer treatment has a habit of being like that, uncomfortable treatment followed by a lull, but not for too long. Like rest breaks in fitness training, you never get quite long enough before you have to start again. This time I was strangely calm. Nothing was a surprise. I was not constantly having to deal with new and scary situations. Dr Ellington and Dr Dawson were performing the surgery. I trusted them and now I had experience of their work. I was far less wound up and anxious. In surgical terms this was nothing compared with my previous operation. The nurses welcomed me back.

'Oh, we thought you were blonde' one of them told me, admiring the black fuzz that was delicately covering my head. I must have looked strange and washed out without hair and eyebrows. This time my roommate was a lovely, chatty lady from the country. She reassured her family all in turn that she was fine, they hadn't done anything yet. Her tumour was benign, but even so I realised how different, and how difficult, it would be to go through this with dependants, children or a partner, relying on you. It was good to talk to her, rather than sitting and worrying in anticipation of the morrow. I wasn't even too phased by the young and nervous resident who arrived later that evening to take my blood sample. 'I'm terribly tired' he told me. 'I don't know if I'm going to be able to get a vein. I'm not good at this.'

'I'm sure you'll be fine' I reassured him, resigning myself to the fact that I was going to emerge with an arm like a pincushion.

This time I do remember going down to theatre. It was very cold and the anaesthetics team were all pale, quiet people. I longed for Dr McCullen with the red socks to introduce some cheer and warm things up. I awoke with some tubes up my nose. I wonder how far up they go? I thought, and promptly went back to sleep. I awoke again briefly to see my friend Dominique, brave enough to come back to visit me despite her fainting episode the previous time.

'Hello Dom' I murmured, reaching out my hand to her, but falling asleep before I touched her. Was she really here I wondered, waking again and finding that she had gone. Nick was glad I was back in hospital. He was able to have his daily feed of hospital fodder. There had to be some benefits for somebody. In fact hospital food was not too bad for me this time; having lost my sense of smell through my first operation I was beginning to learn that there was an upside to my lack of taste. This time I was up and around much sooner. My face was swollen like a watermelon and I had a bulb of fluid from the wound pinned like an emblem on my nightie, but in spite of these I was out of bed and moving. I had had enough of playing the invalid. It is not a role that I had aspired to and it was ill-suited to my impatient temperament. Every morning I would badger the doctors when they were on their rounds.

'Can I go home today?'

More than anything I craved a decent night's sleep. In the end Dr Dawson turned round and told me 'No you can't. You've just had a major operation. You can't go home for several more days.'

So I was stuck there. I listened to Dr Dawson as he made his rounds, talking to his colleagues and to other patients. This man stood out from the other doctors I had met as a natural communicator. He was able to adapt his style very fluidly to suit the situation, pitching the content of his discussions perceptively I thought, as I listened to his conversation with my neighbour (it was not just pure nosiness, there was no way of avoiding overhearing in a hospital ward). He took a lot of time to explain things in terms that each of his patients would understand. I could observe how differently they and their relatives would respond. I am sure that many doctors do not appreciate what a significant difference their individual styles make to their professional interactions. I doubt that Dr Dawson appreciated how effectively he was using his skills.

Once again my friends were fantastic. They continued coming in to spend time with me, when I'm sure they were as fed up with hospitals as I was. I was constantly cheered by their visits and phone calls. There was just one visit that I found was unhelpful and upsetting. A work colleague who was himself quite involved with alternative therapies had arrived one evening. No sooner had he seated himself than he began to tell me how his clairvoyant had told him that it was totally up to me whether I lived or not. He continued to impress on me the virtues of re-birthing, emphasising how critical it was that I took responsibility for my disease and curing it. I tried to defend myself but ended up just bursting into tears. Couldn't he see how helpless I was? I was tired, swollen and tender. I was attached to a drip in a hospital bed. I was a captive audience, I had to listen to him. Even if I was interested in re-birthing this was hardly the ideal setting to discuss it. I was also not in the frame of mind to be told that my recovery was totally down to me so I had better kick myself into action. I had certainly not chosen to put myself through these experiences. Eventually he left. I laid in bed thinking how insensitive he had been. But while I began feeling angry and wondering how he could be so stupid, I had to recognise that, however misguided his comments, the motivation had been a genuine desire to help me. Just like friends who prayed for me he was using his own belief system to try to cure me. I just wished that he had picked his time more carefully.

I got to talk to Leuline, my neighbour, quite a lot. You have so little privacy in hospital that you quickly get to know your neigh-bours well. I believe that we were both able to help each other. I was impressed by the strength that she displayed to her husband and children and, from her descriptions of her life to me, how well she had managed for her family. I don't know what I was able to do for her, but when she left she turned to me and thanked me. 'Thank you for your strength' she had said. I didn't know what strength she had been able to get from me, but I felt that somehow my stay in hospital was justified, not just for myself but that it had had some purpose for somebody else. Maybe it took the edge off some of the feelings of helplessness and dependence that go hand in hand with a hospital stay.

As the days went on, the drips and drains were duly removed. Some were relatively painless, but the drain certainly was not. The nurse arrived in our room one afternoon. It was time to remove both our drains. Who was first? Leuline gamely volunteered. I heard movements behind the curtain, but not a sound did she make. For this occasion I thank her for being strong for me. Nick had arrived just as the nurse had turned her attention to me. 'You may not want to watch this' I warned him. I was glad that he hadn't. Involuntary tears ran down my cheeks as the encrusted drain had tugged on my flesh and started uncoiling as it was pulled out of my neck, like a slithering snake. It hurt like hell.

I was so desperate to get out of hospital that, on the morning of my discharge. I had been up, dressed and packed long before Kev arrived to pick me up. I was out of the door as soon as I saw him walking down the corridor, without even remembering to pick up my drugs and discharge note. He drove me back through the park so that I could see the trees, just to remind me of the nicer things in life. I had had enough of white hospital walls for a while, it was so refreshing to feast my eyes on the expanse of green grass and blue sky. No more hospital beds, at least the next stage would be out-patient treatment.

CHAPTER 6

Tattoos and technology – radiotherapy

Although I had always known that radiotherapy would come at the tail end of my treatment, I really had very little idea what it actually involved. I imagined that it was pretty much like an X-ray. I had read all the leaflets with titles such as 'Radiotherapy – what it means for you' and found their noddy style of writing did little to enhance my understanding. I already knew that I would see a radiotherapist, that I would have the rays administered by a machine and that there were lots of nasty side effects.

'How does it actually work?' I'd asked Dr Newbury.

'If I knew that I wouldn't be here, I'd be lying on a beach somewhere' he helpfully informed me.

'How does it work?' I asked Dr Haxell, recounting my experience with Dr Newbury.

'Well in a way he is right' he replied. 'We really don't quite know how radiation treatment works. It's hard to explain to a lay person, but basically it causes chemical changes as the cells divide.' I began to realise that, despite my need for information and answers, there were some things I would have to take on faith. I would have to accept having radiation shot in to my head without understanding exactly what it was going to do.

'I think that you will find that radiation actually makes you feel worse than the surgery' Dr Haxell told me. 'It will make you feel very tired and depressed. The only good thing is that these effects will begin to get better quite quickly after the treatment has finished.'

So it was like standing on a drawing pin just to feel the relief when you actually get off it. Hopefully it wouldn't really happen to me. There must be some patients who were an exception to the rule. I was a pretty positive person, I'd probably be fine. Dr Newbury expanded on the side effects of the treatment.

'You will feel nauseous, your skin will become irritated and may burn, you will have ulceration down one side of your mouth which may make eating and drinking difficult. You may have some jowling on the right hand side of your face which could be permanent. Your nose will dry up and you will experience crusting as the cells which moisturise your nose are killed by the radiation. You will lose your hair in patches. As the rays pass through your head, a small amount will not be absorbed and will pass straight through your head. These levels are quite safe and will not harm the brain. The hair, however, is a highly sensitive structure and will therefore fall out. This hair loss should be temporary but you may find that you have a small patch of permanent hair loss.'

He paused to let me digest the information he had given me. I ran my hand through my new, baby soft curls. I had only just got used to having hair again and now it was going to fall out. I hoped, unrealistically, that it would only be a tiny patch.

'There are some other possible side effects that I should mention. These are not likely but I have had patients to whom these things have happened.'

He picked up a skull, having understood my need for information.

'Here is your pituitary gland. It controls hormonal function and energy levels. Your tumour was very close to it. We have to treat the area of your tumour plus a margin around it to make sure that we get it all. There is a chance that the radiation could affect the function of your pituitary gland. We can deal with that if it happens. Now, the other problem is here' he gestured, 'the optic nerve.'

He traced its path.

'I had one patient, a long time ago, who did actually go blind. It is highly unlikely but there is a slim chance that that could happen.'

These risks were very small. I decided to dismiss them. They wouldn't happen to me, I decided. There had been a 10% chance of me having an epileptic fit and I hadn't so why should I go blind or experience disrupted pituitary function? It was an interesting way of looking at percentage risks. When, at the time of my diagnosis, I had believed that I may only have a 10% chance of a cure I had convinced myself that I would be in that 10%. I had focused on all the times I had taken exams or been in sporting events and come in the top 10%. I had done everything to make that 10% seem realistically possible. Now I was doing the reverse. 10% became minimal, shrinking away into insignificance until it no longer seemed worth considering. Later, I met a fellow patient in the hospital, a man in his early thirties who had just been diagnosed with a brain tumour. The doctors had recommended surgery but, when explaining the risks, had warned that there was a 10% risk of paralysis down one side of his body. 'That is too much' he had told me in anguish. 'I just couldn't deal with the thought of being partially paralysed.' I'd asked him what he would do. 'Just have the radiotherapy' he had replied. His prognosis was poor and he believed his chances of survival were slim. I wondered how specific the doctors had been with that 10% figure. I had been quoted 10% by Dr Jarman and 5% by his registrar as the chances of experiencing an epileptic fit. Did they just mean 'a very small chance', did they mean with all the surgeons performing this procedure or with their own team operating? We all pick numbers out of the air to indicate risks as non-specific as small, medium or large. Once we use numbers our estimates take on an unwarranted but mystical scientific significance. Would the man with the brain tumour have responded differently if he had been told there was a 5% chance, and maybe decided to have the surgery that would have given him a better chance at life?

Once Dr Newbury had explained the side effects and their associated risks that were relevant to me he explained that they needed to measure me up for the treatment. I was sent down to the basement and into the hands of the technicians. I was required to lie on a metal bed underneath a large machine. I lay still, as instructed, as they tried to position my head. I was obviously causing some difficulties, but I wasn't sure what because no one spoke to me.

'Try her on a polystyrene mattress' someone suggested.

I took this as a cue to get off the bed, the 'her' was obviously referring to me, as they rearranged the set up. On I got again and the nameless technician fiddled around for a while.

'We're going to put a mask on you' someone told me.

Suddenly, a hot, damp sheet was slapped over my face. I couldn't see and breathing was more difficult. I panicked internally, I felt very claustrophobic. It brought back all the memories of the first MRI scan I had had. Breathe deeply, I told myself. It won't be too long. If you move you'll only ruin it and they'll have to start all over again. They began drawing on my face, taking measurements from my ears and making gentle adjustment to the position of my head.

'We're going to take a film now' a voice came out of my blackness.

I was left in silence. I waited, for what seemed like an eternity, but was probably no more than six or seven minutes. Where was everybody? I made a muffled sound through the mask and tapped the bed with my hands in the hope of catching someone's attention.

'Oh, are you all right?' Someone entered the room, remembering that I was still there. 'The films aren't right. We're going to have to do it again' the voice continued. 'Can't you put your head back further?'

I tried pushing the back of my head down, aided uncomfortably by the owner of the voice pushing on my forehead, to no avail. The mask was removed.

'You're going to have to get your head back further' I was crossly informed.

'I can't' I apologised, feeling that I was being deliberately obstructive. My neck was still very swollen and there was no flexibility to move it any further. Trying to force it was causing shooting pains through my ear. 'I really can't get it back any further, I'm sorry.' They tried again, a different mattress, no mask, but there wasn't a solution. They were getting more and more impatient. Didn't they realise that I was more keen than anybody to get this over and done with and get the treatment underway? Several films later they gave up. Dr Newbury appeared and explained that they had to get the bone at the base of the eye socket vertical. They needed to treat around the eye without getting the eye itself so the angle needed to be exact. I was glad that he was being so precise. He hoped that the swelling would have reduced enough to enable my head to reach the appropriate position by the following week. I went back home to wait.

The experience had shaken me. I reasoned that it was probably because the whole thing was so technical. I had felt like part of the machinery, with people talking about me as if I wasn't there. It was as if I were a car on an assembly line, every technician doing their own bit with little understanding of the finished product. Dr Haxell asked me how it had gone. I told him, explaining how alienating I had found the experience.

'I guess they're so busy with dealing with the technical things that they haven't really got time to explain what's going on' I finished.

'That's no excuse' he replied sharply, 'it's their job to deal with patients. They should not make you feel like that.'

I thought maybe they didn't realise how I had felt. So the next time I went back I thought I would tell them.

'It's very alienating with a mask on, not being able to see and not understanding what's going on' I told them. 'Would you mind telling me when you're doing something, and explaining what's happening?'

'Of course not' they agreed.

I felt far less isolated. They talked the whole way through and were constantly checking that I was all right.

This time they got it right. My head was sufficiently flexed and they were able to take the required films. I was astounded by the amount of measuring and checking that was required. My head was taped to the table as I lay on my back, a band across my forehead to prevent any undesirable movement. Tattoos were injected on to both sides of my head. They wanted to put one on my upper lip but I objected.

'Doesn't my face look strange enough already?' I asked miserably.

So they settled for a permanent ink dot under my nose. I also had the perimeter of the radiation fields marked on to my chest and neck. I looked like I had spent hours covering myself in war paint. It was only six weeks I told myself, then I could scrub them off.

'Now be careful not to wash them off' they warned me, 'otherwise we'll have to do them all over again.' I was certain I wouldn't. I had no wish to repeat the performance.

My radiation treatment was scheduled to start for real the following week. I had been instructed to turn up early for the first session as it would take a little longer to set up. By chance, my friend Daniel had the afternoon off. He offered to accompany me, and thereby unfortunately forfeited the rest of his afternoon. Daniel happily made friends with most of the radiotherapy department staff and could tell me the majority of their life stories by the time I was finished. Arriving at the appropriate machine I was introduced to the radiotherapy team and shown through into a large, spacious room. The walls were an orangey pink colour, like a flavourless tropical sorbet. Leaning my head against the wall I discovered that the walls were covered in a soft material. The centrepiece of the room was a large machine overhanging a metal bed. Stacked neatly in the corner of the room were several different mattresses and the shelves held a series of clamps not dissimilar to those I remembered from school chemistry labs. I was instructed to lie face up on the bed with my head hanging over the edge of the mattress. My head was then adjusted to an appropriate position using masking tape. I stared up into what I saw as the eye of the machine, seeing my own eyes reflected back. Once again there was an incredible amount of measuring. Would you get obsessed by measuring in this job? Did overwrought radiologists break out into a quantifying mania, a frenzy of measuring everything that moved? I thought back to a brief period of my life when I had, as a student of civil engineering, been sent on a surveying course. Standing in the rain with theodolites was not my idea of fun. I'd made a series of rough and ready estimates of angles, assuring the boys that I was working with 'I'm sure that will do'. I was glad that the radiologists appeared to have a greater penchant for detail than I had demonstrated by my own slap-dash approach.

In order to minimise the damage that the radiation would cause to healthy tissues it would, they informed me, be necessary to shield out a number of structures, including my right eye and my mouth, with thick lead weights. These were suspended over my face by clamps. Precise templates needed to be drawn to ensure that the blocks were in the same place for all thirty of the treatments that I would have. Once again I felt quite uninvolved in the process. One of the radiologists, a young guy called Simon, would chat to me as they worked, explaining what was going on, telling me about his uncle in England and making the pair of us seem human. The others were engrossed in the technical aspects of their work. It must have been like a production line for them, with so many patients coming through each day, but I appreciated those small interactions that differentiated me from part of the machinery.

Once the setting up was completed they could press the start button and we were ready to begin. The actual treatment process was amazingly quick, seconds in fact. A total of twenty minutes each day, and most of that was setting up time. I lay with a pillow underneath my knees and my hands clutching the edge of the pillow to keep my shoulders flat down and motionless. My head was taped to the table so that, for once in my life, I was still. The lead blocks were lined up with the proforma of shadows that they had drawn up. I was instructed to keep looking back at a reel of tape that had been suspended like a pendulum from the machine and circled hypnotically. Everyone would vanish from the room and there would be a loud buzzing over the radio that was playing. The buzzing stopped and the door immediately clicked open. They were straight back in, reorganising blocks and angles for the next zap. There were three in all. The second through the side of my neck and the third slightly lower, treating the lymph node area of my neck. I got used to the routine. I would switch off my mind for the time that I was in there, blankly watching the pendulum swing. It helped me deal with the alienating situation I had found myself propelled into.

I was rudely awoken from my day dreaming on one occasion. Staring up blankly at the ceiling I suddenly saw the clamp and a large lead weight falling towards my face – it seemed to fall in slow motion, allowing me to focus on its hard contours before it struck. My head was firmly taped to the table, I could do nothing but watch. The radiotherapists panicked. They rushed to untape me, apologising profusely. Was I OK? Bruised or bleeding? Stunned? Concussed? It really hadn't hurt that much. I was fine, just fine, I assured them. It was only when they had handed me some tissues that I realised that there were tears running down my face. It must have been a shock reaction, but illustrated perfectly how helpless I felt, I couldn't even protect myself from objects falling on my face. The radiotherapy team insisted that I see a doctor but I really was all right. The bruising was internal and psychological.

A couple of months later I realised that my experience with the lead blocks, well mixed with the MRI scans, had made an interesting cocktail. They had compounded to make me claustrophobic. I panicked if I felt that I was trapped and I hated not being able to move. I was by now familiar with the physical reactions connected with my panic attacks. A friend and I had visited an art gallery where the prime attraction was a maze in the pitch black. You would have to feel your way through, using your sense of touch as your guide, robbed of your vision. The whole thing took as little as five minutes to negotiate yourself through. The squeals and giggles of the other explorers enticed me in. I had been in the cavernous blackness for less than 30 seconds when I began to feel my breathing tightening. The metal bands were back in place. It was the first panic attack I had had in months. I had to get out. Focusing hard on my breathing, I backtracked and to my relief got myself back to the entrance. I felt so stupid, after all it was only a maze, but to me there was nothing fun about experiencing that feeling of helplessness all over again.

As with the chemotherapy, there was no way to tell whether the radiotherapy was actually working but I was experiencing the side effects all right. My mouth was badly ulcerated and I was feeling pretty nauseous. I had a diet that largely consisted of bananas, yoghurt and custard. I feared that I was in severe danger of turning yellow. It was several months before I could face bananas again, and banana custard is certainly off the menu. I found that the radiation was blocking the tear ducts to my right eye and my eye was constantly weeping. Then my hair began falling out. I had gone to stay with my sister in Adelaide for the weekend. I went with hair and came back with two big gaping squares, one on the top of my head and one on the back. I couldn't fathom out how they had appeared. I'd understood that I would lose the hair on the back of my head as the rays passed through it, but how had I managed to lose the hair on the top? I imagined the rays refracting off some internal object and making a 90 degree turn up towards the sky. I asked one of the radiographers. She thought for a moment. 'We tie your head back at an angle, so the rays are not going directly through your face but are in fact directed upwards, parallel with your forehead.' Problem solved, in one way. More practically I was back to wearing hats. I faced a dilemma. Previously I had shaved my head but now I had a scar from ear to ear, being bald was not going to be the solution. I decided to keep the patches. Some hair was warmer than none and I liked having hair.

During my six weeks of radiotherapy I had regular appointments with the doctors. Sometimes I saw Dr Newbury but, more often than not, it was Dr Connolly, his registrar. Dr Connolly was a young woman, graceful and quietly spoken. She was one of those doctors who had chosen to specialise in oncology because she was obviously extremely compassionate. She would talk quite slowly and make a lot of eye contact. Her kindness and concern were sincere. I found her both honest and understanding. She would always give a straight answer to my questions, even if the answer was not particularly what I wanted to hear. She helped me deal with my side effects in a practical but sympathetic way. She did not, like some doctors, acknowledge the symptoms I described with 'Yes of course, but I did warn you that this would happen', but began empathetically 'You poor thing, that must be uncomfortable. There is something that you could do about that.' I found that I was asking to see or speak to Dr Connolly rather than Dr Newbury if there was a problem. It was simply far easier to relate to her. She took time to answer my questions and did not make me feel like my side effects were trivial. I had the feeling that some oncologists were very interested in treating the actual disease but felt that in comparison the side effects were almost trivial. After all, they were saving your life, weren't they? You should just shut up and put up. It is far easier for a patient to remain amenable and positive if they are not experiencing discomfort. And, after all, quality of life is a predictor of quantity of life, and my side effects certainly impacted upon my quality of life.

Radiation treatment has a cumulative effect. I started off hoping that I was going to be one of the lucky ones, that Dr Haxell would be wrong and I would not experience the lethargy, tiredness and depression. After a few weeks I discovered, once again, that I was not an exception, he was quite correct. I was exhausted. If I lay down in the middle of the day I would fall straight into a heavy sleep. I gave up my medication because every time I tried to do it I would be drifting off. I had avoided watching TV during my illness. I am not much of a TV watcher and could think of better things to do with my time. Now I just didn't have the energy or inclination to think of anything more creative to do. I became an avid watcher of American talk shows and exhausted the supply at the local video shop. I had a chart on my desk and was counting off the days until my treatment finished. My skin was beginning to burn on the back of my neck and red patches appeared on my face. The treatment was taking its toll. Dr Haxell's daughter, who was pregnant at the time, was a wonderful support to me. She regularly took me to the hospital for my daily dose. I enjoyed her company, she had some interesting ideas and a lot of warmth and kindness. In a strange way I drew an analogy between our experiences, cancer was rather like being pregnant. A prolonged waiting period associated with constant body and life style changes, and, like any major life change, it triggered a fresh and critical look at values and priorities.

And then it was my birthday. Near the end of my radiotherapy I had something to celebrate. At one time I had wondered whether I would live to be 26. Here I was, a little bruised and battered but I was most certainly still here. Friends arranged a weekend away horse riding. We rented a country cottage and cooked a traditional Christmas meal. Turkey, Christmas pudding, the works. I tried to numb my mouth ulcers with champagne, but they stung awfully. Still it didn't dampen my birthday spirits. Although the final stretch, the radiotherapy, was not the happiest time of my life, it did have its positive moments.

Radiotherapy being a daily occurrence, I met a number of the other regulars. Two of them particularly stuck in my mind. One was a young boy, maybe 12 or 13. He would appear every morning accompanied by one of his parents. As he had his treatment I would chat to his father. He had had a tumour four years before and they had hoped that it was long gone, but then it recurred, this time in his lung. They were unsure of his chances. The boy was so mature about his disease. He appeared to be fully aware of his condition and the treatments involved. He would talk about the side effects that he was experiencing and how tired the radiotherapy was making him feel, but sometimes he was dressed in his school uniform so he was obviously managing a bit of school. It must have been desperately hard for the whole family. It made me a little more aware of the stress, anxiety and helplessness that must be experienced by a parent whose child is sick. I had maybe not been fully appreciative of how difficult it must be for my parents. I had felt that I could not deal with their emotions and fears as well as my own and had encouraged them to find support elsewhere.

The other individual who made a lasting impression was a man in his mid-thirties. He was always cheery and pleasant to be around. I discovered that he was in the army. He was always at the hospital alone. I wondered who he had to support him. He told me his story, complete with the emotions. There is sometimes an amazing honesty between complete strangers in waiting rooms. He had had a painful elbow; resting it and physiotherapy had achieved nothing. Eventually one of the army surgeons had operated. They had found a tumour that may have been present for up to ten years. The army doctors had quickly referred him to the hospital where the doctors had recommended that they amputate his arm. That would give him the optimal chance of survival they had told him. He was trying to come to terms with the idea. He had been looking into prosthetics and what they could manage to do with them these days. Through his shock he was trying to find some practical solutions, to make the whole process more manageable. His entire life would change radically. A soldier is not much use with only one arm. He was looking at huge life changes. I hoped that he would be able to deal with them. He seemed to be rational and brave, but after all he was army trained. I was often struck, throughout my treatments, by the openness and honesty with which people discussed their diseases. There were incredible examples of strength, determination and bravery displayed by some of the individuals I met. It was, at times, quite humbling.

I had always maintained that I wanted to have all my treatment in Australia, that going back to England would be like giving up. I was not going to give up and I could get through this on my own. The less energy I had, the more I wanted to go home. I was in desperate need of a holiday. I had booked a flight for a month or so after the radiation treatment finished, having convinced myself that I would be fine by then. A couple of weeks to get worse and then a couple of weeks to recover. My hair might even be growing back by then I reasoned. As each day wore slowly by I found myself growing more and more homesick. I somehow believed that everything would be all right if I could get home. I needed a pair of ruby slippers to get back to Auntie Em.

I had said that when I finished my treatment I would throw a massive party to thank all my friends for the love and support they had given me throughout the nine months of my illness. Now it came to it I couldn't think of anything worse. I had a little brunch with Dr Haxell's daughter down at the beach, hot in the warm winter sun. I had given myself 48 hours to pack my bags and get my plane. I was laden with requests for things English, M&S underwear, tinned custard, Marmite and cider. All the things that ex-pat friends were missing from home. A friend drove me to the airport. As we sat drinking coffee I looked out of the window. Would I come back here again? I had a return ticket, booked for six weeks time but I just didn't know. When I boarded the plane I felt that I was escaping, that my recovery had begun.

CHAPTER 7

England's pastures green – coming home

Travelling alone restored a sense of capability and independence to me. I was anonymous to everybody on that plane. No one knew that I had had cancer, I was just a young woman in a hat with a swollen face. Luckily my neighbour did not want to converse. I took a couple of sleeping pills and was awoken by the announcement that we would soon be arriving in Hong Kong.

I had been in Hong Kong a couple of years before. It had been my first stop on my outward trip. The contrast between trips was as marked as that of the blue harbour and beaches of Sydney with the city lights and neon of my new surroundings. Last time I had been here I had been full of energy, beginning an adventure, excited by the world that I was about to explore. I had been so young and free. Now it's a hectic buzz that just made me tired. I sought the solace of the business lounge and stuck my nose into a book. I didn't want to have to process the new and invading stimuli, I wanted to be encased in a translucent bubble so that nothing else could touch me, so that I was safe and alone. I tucked myself away in a corner, my book hiding my face, only vaguely aware of the myriad planes, randomly touching down and taking off. Soon it was time for the second leg of the journey. I was back in a similar plane seat, eating similar food, watching similar films and taking the same sleeping tablets. It was a painless and drowsy journey, until we crossed the south coast of England.

I wriggled to the window, peering intently at the emerging ground below. Where exactly were we? I tried to pinpoint our position on the coast. I breathed in the view, sucking it deep into my memory. The patchwork fields that welcome every English person home. The familiar greens and browns, the square brown homes like monopoly houses, the toy cars and the telegraph poles. As we neared Heathrow and began our descent they got nearer, the details more precise, a black cab and a red bus. I felt the prickle of tears beginning in my eyes. I was coming home. For the first time in my life it actually felt like home. Awaiting my luggage, I approached the nearby exchange kiosk to change some money. I was delighted by the ten pound notes. 'They're so pale' I exclaimed. I was so pleased to see English money again. The lady behind the counter gave me a quizzical look. She probably had all sorts of strange people passing through, I was just another rather disorientated passenger who thought all British things were quaint.

Airport trolleys are on a par with shopping trolleys and the supposedly transportable hospital machines. I wended my way through the formalities of passports and customs. We arrived at exactly the same time, my old friends and I. There were lots of tears and hugging. It seemed so little time since I had seen them, yet another life had happened to me in between. I hugged them tight. It was good to be home.

I had intended to come home for a six week holiday. There were so many people I wanted to see and so much to catch up on. I was also incredibly tired. My energy reserves were in the red and a warning light was flashing. After a couple of weeks I was exhausted. I was telling the same story over and over again, anxious that my friends and family should understand. I was also disappointed that my side effects, rather than rapidly abating as I had optimistically hoped, were getting worse. My face was badly swollen, the burn marks on my skin were more pronounced and my nasal problems worsening. I was also under some pressure to make a decision to come back home and stay here. Family and friends who had been unable to be present during my illness understandably wanted to help me to recuperate. Stay here, they urged me. Naomi, having come home for a holiday, had decided that, as much as she loved Australia, she was English and that this was her home. She also wanted me to stay. I had also had the long awaited face-to-face reunion with my natural mother. Hugging her as we met, I did not feel that I was meeting a stranger. Originally invited to lunch, I had ended up staying for dinner too. I wanted to give this relationship a chance to develop, to get to know my half brother and sister. That would be hard to do from the other side of the world. The more old friends I saw, the more my roots were tugging at me. I didn't know what to do. Deciding that I was not in a fit state of mind to make a decision, I decided to make a temporary one. I would stay here for a while and take the next step once I felt ready. Any decision I made feeling so despondent and low would undoubtedly be wrong.

My side effects eventually drove me to a GP. He reacted in horror when I told him what I had had. He could not help with the side effects, he confessed, he knew little about my disease. He recommended that I contact a specialist. So I was to begin my encounter with the British medical system. My first problem was who to contact and where. Dr Newbury had told me that if I had any problems while I was away I should contact Dr Fraser at one of the London hospitals. I called to make an appointment. The first problem was a referral. I went back to the GP's practice and saw a different doctor, Dr Ayling. Dr Ayling was young, probably about my own age, and very easy to talk to. 'Don't worry' she assured me. 'I'll do the referral and you arrange for the notes to be sent over from Australia.' That sounded pretty straightforward.

It wasn't. Contacting Australia to request my notes was fine, but attending my hospital appointment a week later I found they were in a state of confusion. I did not see the consultant I was expecting but his registrar Dr Bailey. Unsure what my problem was he had roped in an ENT guy, Mr Carroll. They only knew that I had 'some nasal problem' and hadn't a clue about the treatment that I had had. No notes had arrived. I couldn't understand it. I had provided a fax number and appointment date to Australia. Why hadn't the information arrived? They decided they'd better check things out themselves. Once again I had an endoscopy. This one was attached to a large TV screen so that all in the room could see. Naomi and I watched with interest as they conducted a guided tour of the inside of my nose. Everything appeared to be fine, no obvious tumour returning. It was difficult for them to deal with my side effects and questions without any notes. 'Come back for a CT scan' they requested, 'hopefully we should have your notes by then.' The scan was scheduled for a couple of weeks time. As we drove home I considered the consultation. They had all been very pleasant and willing to help but, without notes there was little they could do. I called Sydney and requested the urgent transfer of my notes.

Before the date of my scheduled CT scan I noticed that my face was swelling again. Erratically it seemed to go up and down with a will of its own. It was uncomfortable and made me conscious about my face, exacerbating my facial bruising, it was obviously visible. People would ask me in the street 'What happened? Have you been in a fight?' Maybe once they had my notes in they would be able to help me. I rang the hospital to talk to Dr Bailey. Dr Bailey was away I was informed, they would try someone else. The phone went blank. 'Hello', I checked to see that it had.

Silence. I began to talk, explaining who I was trying to contact and why.

'He is not here' the heavily accented voice told me. 'Would you explain what is the problem to me?' I hesitated, would this person understand? Her English was very bad.

I explained about my face, how it would swell up so uncomfortably, and then a few days later start subsiding again. I couldn't understand why, I wondered could they help me? The voice considered it for a while.

'I cannot tell without looking at you what is this thing. You can come in tomorrow, yes? OK, bye.'

'Hold on, what time?' I rushed before the phone cut off.

'10.00, OK? Bye,' the phone went dead.

I had to go in for a CT scan anyway, so assuming that it was the clinic that I had attended before, I could do both at one time.

My father drove me up to the hospital armed with a briefcase full of work as he was anticipating a long wait. We arrived at the outpatient clinic where I was surprised to find that they had no idea that I was coming. No appointment had been booked.

'Who did you speak to?' the receptionist asked me as I explained the story.

I didn't know. The voice had never identified itself.

'Well she was foreign' I started unhelpfully, 'maybe German?' I guessed wildly and inaccurately. 'I ended up speaking to her when I tried to contact Dr Bailey.'

'We'll try to find out' she told me. 'Take a seat.'

We waited and waited. I began to worry that I would miss my scan. I explained to the receptionist that I had other appointments, that I couldn't wait all morning without upsetting the scanning timetable. Should I leave and come back? We were in the midst of debating a solution when one of the sisters arrived. She'd tracked down 'the voice'. She showed me through.

The voice, it turned out, belonged to a large Brazilian woman who was filling in for Dr Bailey.

'Please excuse me, I am not yet so good with the language' she began.

Well presumably she was au fait with the medical aspects of her job. She felt my face. 'Do you get much pouss?' she asked me.

'I beg your pardon, I don't understand you.'

'Do you get much pouss?' she repeated.

I stared blankly, my mind trying to figure out what she was talking about. What was pouss?

'Have I not got the right word?' she asked me, grasping that I did not understand.

'Pouss, P U S,' now I got it.

'No, none' I told her. I was getting impatient. There had been no appointment and now I was getting no answers because I couldn't understand the questions. I am all for international training and the sharing of expertise that it engenders, but for the patients' and the doctors' sakes a certain level of fluent conversational English is essential.

'So why does it happen?'

'Well it just happens' she told me, shrugging her shoulders.

'No one told me that it would be a consequence of my treatment' I continued. 'I need to understand why it happens, whether I can do anything for it, how long it will last for.'

'I cannot explain it' she told me.

Did she mean she didn't know or that she could only explain to me in Portuguese?

'Come back tomorrow and I will find someone who can tell you.'

I left in a rush to have my scans.

'She probably knew what she was talking about' I complained to my Dad, 'but she certainly couldn't communicate it to me.'

The CT scan and chest X-ray were quickly over. I sat in the car disgruntled all the way home. Maybe they would be able to help me tomorrow. It was probably very difficult me arriving as a patient having been treated overseas, not being in the system and not having built up a relationship with a consultant in this country that I could talk to. It could have been my own fault, maybe I should have asked more questions about the side effects before the radiation and anticipated this happening. Should it happen? Was it normal?

The next morning my friend Izzy phoned.

'How did it go at the hospital yesterday?'

I told her the saga.

'I've got to go back today' I finished off. 'Hopefully they can tell me what is happening this time. I wish someone would just tell me what happens next, what the ongoing situation is.'

I was beginning to feel very lost. Once again I had no idea of what the future held in terms of medical checks, when I would begin to feel better again and when the side effects would vanish.

'Why is it so hard?' I lamented to Izzy, 'why can't someone just tell me what is going to happen?'

'Who's coming with you today?' she asked.

'Oh, I'm going on my own, but it'll be fine' I assured her.

'No you're not. What time is your appointment? I'm jumping in a cab and I'll see you there.' She hung up.

I was glad that she came as I was beginning to feel very vulnerable and tired, I was finding it difficult to try to manage the medical system. I was relieved to have her company and support. My Brazilian registrar of the previous day had drafted in Mr Carroll. Mr Carroll was relaxed and approachable. I was glad to see him. I started to explain about my face.

'Before we talk about that I've got some results for you' he reminded me, flicking through the notes. He seemed to take an age just turning pages. I sat forward expectantly.

'Your CT was clear and' he turned another page, 'your X-ray was clear too.'

He grinned at me, I smiled back at hime and then at Iz.

'That's good isn't it' she confirmed.

It was more than good, it was brilliant. My first follow-up scan and I was clear. I turned my attentions to my face. Was it an allergy, my mother's cat or dog? Unlikely, Mr Carroll thought. He could give me some nasal spray just in case. It could be a condition connected with unequal pressure in capillaries, which he dutifully explained in detail, but it may well just be a result of the radiation and the surgery. He really wasn't sure. His difficulties were compounded by the fact that they still had not received the full details of my treatment.

'We have the information about your surgery and your chemotherapy from the radiotherapy department who compiled this report, but they have neglected to give any details as regards your radiation treatment' he informed me. 'We'll have to chase it up.'

I was used to a business world where international communication was a daily occurrence, by phone, fax, e-mail, couriers, video conferencing. My world was a high tech place. How could it take more than a month to transfer a few pieces of paper? I was astounded that I would have to ring Sydney again.

Mr Carroll continued. People don't usually complain about the swelling a year or so later, he assured me. Maybe they had just got used to it, he hypothesised. But I did not want to wait a 'year or so'. I wanted a solution.

'You could go and see Dr Broderick' he suggested. 'He may be able to help you.' More appointments, more maybes. I knew they were trying to help but the appointment was a long while away and my face was sore. Every day I would wake up and prod it cautiously, feeling gently around my jawbone to see if I could feel the bone through the turgid flesh that covered it. Days when I could were good days, my neck and shoulders were less stiff from the tension. I was disappointed when it seemed more swollen and would check the mirror regularly to identify any visible changes as the day progressed. In the end I got fed up with looking at my battered face and draped a scarf over my mirror. I'd stick to gauging its progress by touch.

As Izzy and I sat in the pharmacy waiting for my drugs I began to talk, spilling all the anxieties and frustrations that had been slowly building up inside. I found every trip to the hospital difficult. Every consultation was a reaffirmation of my ongoing nightmare. Combined with the changes of moving country, staying for a while with my mother, the difficult family interactions, organising with the firm to rejoin the UK practice and ship my belongings back to England. There was too much going on. I felt unable to cope and I would find myself bursting into tears at the slightest provocation. Every minor issue turned into major stress. Particularly with my family. I was not easy to live with and I found it difficult trying to deal with pent up concerns that they had been unable to share with me while I was in Sydney. I was missing the established day-to-day support I had from friends in Australia, the objective outlet I had had from talking to Andrew. I could only bottle things up for a certain time, now it all came out.

'Come on' said Izzy, 'we're going out for lunch.' She did a lot of the listening while I did most of the talking, about how overwhelmed I felt, how low and depressed, that it was so difficult not knowing how long it would take to get better, being unable to make any plans. Sometimes, I told her, it just all seemed too hard. I wished I was dead so that I no longer had to go on dealing with life and with trying to cope. I was overwhelmed with living and sinking deeper daily, under its weight. I had hit an all time low.

It seemed strange to me that it was when, as others would suggest, 'the worst was over' that I hit a period of such total blackness. The world seemed to be a bleak and hard place, constructed in dull, insipid colours and harsh, twisted materials. My world took on the perspective of a long deserted battlefield, of a hastily evacuated town abandoned to nothingness. My life felt empty. 'There is nothing in my life. I don't know why I just didn't die. I don't want to have to be alive' I had sobbed one night, trying to explain to my mother how I felt. If I had not fought so hard for my life there were times when I believe I could have ended it.

I believe the hospital could have and should have done something to help me, but there was no one consistent to manage my case. No one ever asked me how I was feeling, that was left to the company doctor at work. I saw Dr Withall at the recommendation of my wise and wonderful personnel manager, herself a cancer survivor, who advised that I should have someone objective to talk to. She was right. Dr Withall rapidly dismissed any of my tentative ideas that I should really think about returning to work.

'You're obviously not fit for work' he told me early on in our discussion, 'and won't be for a while', scuppering my plans that anticipated I would be fit and well by the end of the month. It was a weight off my mind. I no longer had to feel guilty that I should be back at work. He listened as I described my story, culminating in my current feelings.

'I was wondering if you knew anyone I could talk to?' I asked, describing the discussions I had had with Andrew. 'My GP suggested a psychiatric nurse who works at their practice but I know that is not what I need, I'm a psychologist myself, I think I know what I need. It was so helpful for me to be able to talk to someone in Sydney who specialised in psycho-oncology.'

'I can definitely recommend someone' he assured me. 'He's excellent. I use him a lot.'

I was relieved that I could begin to build my framework of support. I needed someone who could help me to reflect back on the events of the previous years, to digest, understand and accept them. I had too many pressures and decisions and was trying to deal with too many changes, I needed to sort things out.

'Do you think you might be depressed?' Dr Withall cut in to my thoughts.

'Well, I'm sleeping OK' I began, my thoughts running through the diagnostic criteria, but the way I was feeling was definitely not my normal positive self.

'I guess I could be' I mused. 'I don't really like the idea of antidepressants, I think that cognitive therapy is what I need. It's just all the changes and my home situation that are getting to me.'

'You may like to try some antidepressants' he suggested. 'Talk to your GP about them if you think they would help.'

He didn't push me but just gently planted the seed.

Later that week I was once again in blackness, clouds of tears hanging over my head, preventing me from coping with everyday tasks. I was unable to deal with my shipping arrangements or make my mind up about where to live. I can't go on like this, I wailed to myself, I have to make it stop. I made a snap decision. I may not like the idea of antidepressants but it was not as bad as feeling such overwhelming bleakness. I made an urgent appointment to see my GP, Dr Ayling.

'Frankly' she informed me, 'I'd be surprised if you didn't need them considering what you've been through.' She handed me a prescription. 'Try these and see how you go. I think you'll find they make a difference, but we'll monitor you and see.'

I thought back to the essays I had written at university about antidepressants and their side effects. The beauty of these newer drugs, she told me, was their lack of side effects in most people. For once in my life, as far as side effects go, I was not, unfortunately, most people. The drug I was taking was called 'Lustral'. It turned me into a zombie. I slept for fourteen or fifteen hours a day. When I was awake I was, for all intents and purposes, still absent. I could happily while away the remaining hours staring blankly into space. I had shooting pains through my arms and neck and a constant feeling of sickness.

'Keep trying' the doctor encouraged, 'the symptoms usually disappear after a week or so.' But my symptoms were going nowhere. They had set up camp and sent for reinforcements. I felt awful. After two weeks she too acknowledged that we were defeated. Stop taking them and we'll try you on something else, she advised.

'Surmontil', that was what the printed label said. I hoped that it would work better and work quickly. I needed some relief. A fortnight of side effects had done nothing to boost my psychological morale. Dr Ayling decided to play it safe, she started me on a low dose and began to build it up. She had a lovely consulting style that worked well for me. She remembered me as an individual and would discuss medication in detail so that we could come to a mutual decision about what might work and the side effects that would be acceptable to me. As I upped the dose I began to feel the benefits. I hadn't realised how unlike myself I had been until my personality began to emerge again. I felt my black cloud lift within a week, blown away by a wind of synthetic chemical. I began to have more energy, life was less of a burden and an effort. I began to want to live again.

I spent a week with friends, Jo and Jeff, who had recently moved up to Manchester. They were on the doorsteps of the Peaks and the Lake District. As we walked in this beautiful country I began to stop thinking about cancer, to look forward to my life. I stopped and turned in a circle, looking around me, enjoying being in that exact moment, in that exact spot. As the winds blew over the peaks, it reached through to my core, loosening my bleakness, my frustrations and my fears. The rain beat down, dislodging their hold and washed them away into the valleys and lakes, leaving me free. How could I have wanted to be dead just a few weeks ago? The world was such a wonderful place. Everywhere I looked around me there was life, from the red squirrel, to the hardened sheep, to the autumnal bracken and the trees. I began to feel my old excitement and enthusiasm returning. I could not possibly give up on life, there was so much to do, so much to explore and enjoy, I'd never fit it all in. I relished beginning to regain my physical strength. The walking and cycling reminded me how much pleasure I got from physical exercise, how good it felt to move and stretch my muscles, stretching out the tension of the previous months. Another facet of my personality was being restored, one that helped me deal with stress and depression. It was a timely reunion.

Eventually the appointment with Dr Broderick came to fruition. I attended the specified clinic and, following the customary hospital wait, I was located by a rather confused consultant.

'Sorry to keep you waiting, but we've got your notes and we're trying to work out why you've been referred to us. We know you've been referred from another doctor in this hospital, but we're not sure exactly who or why.'

I should not have been surprised.

'I think it's because you may be able to do something about the swelling in my neck. You see I had a rhabdomyosarcoma...' I told the story again. It was getting very repetitive. Maybe I could liven it up a bit, put it to music and turn it into a song?

He carefully felt around my neck.

'Is there any pattern to its swelling?' he questioned me carefully.

'I can't identify one' I replied, 'it appears to be pretty random. I was worrying that it could be allergies but it doesn't seem to be exacerbated by anything in particular. It subsided initially after the neck dissection but swelled considerably during the radiation.'

'You may well have allergies' he told me, learning that I had asthma and hay fever, 'but I don't think that is what is causing the swelling. It is probably due to the surgery and the radiotherapy. I wonder if some MLD therapy might help you?'

'What is MLD therapy?' I asked fearfully, hoping to avoid further treatment.

'Manual lymphatic drainage therapy. We're just beginning to use it in this country. We don't actually do it here but we could organise for you to have it done privately. One of the sisters will call you to organise it.'

I breathed an internal sigh of relief that the corporate medical insurance covered my treatment costs now that I had returned to England. I had just about run out of cash for alternative or private treatments. It would be such a luxury to have a face that wasn't sore and swollen. Maybe I wouldn't look quite so strange.

I awaited a call. Nothing came. Maybe they'll call next week, but they didn't. In the end I called them.

'I was hoping that one of the sisters would contact me to arrange further treatment' I told Dr Broderick's secretary. Someone would call me back, she assured me. But someone didn't call me back. A week later I called again. I was getting to know the hospital telephone system well. Eventually I got through to a sister.

'Oh, I was going to call you but I haven't had a chance to speak to Dr Broderick. He didn't say anything about organising follow-up treatment to us.'

I explained what he had suggested in my consultation.

'OK, well I'll give you the name of a practitioner and ask Dr Broderick to write a referral letter, now that you're on the phone.'

All I had needed was a letter and a phone number, but it had taken three weeks and two phone calls to get it. If my face had not been so uncomfortable I think I would have given up. How incredibly inefficient this process had been. I didn't know whether it was the people or the system, but from my point of view I wanted help. It was stressful and frustrating to be promised assistance that did not emerge without persistence and pushing. I had suffered the discomfort of a sore face for longer than I needed to. I did not want to be told that it was the doctor's fault, or that the delays had been due to the system. I needed someone to take responsibility for organising the treatment I required, not, however nicely put, apologies and excuses. I wondered how other patients managed to get the treatment they needed. Did they too continually push the system, even the elderly or very ill, or did they eventually accept the lack of forthcoming help and give up?

Although my treatment was over I was still worried about the continuing monitoring I needed. I had no idea what the process would be. How often did I need scans? Did I need scans at all? How would I know if the disease was coming back? Where could it recur? There was no one who I could ask. Every time friends and relatives asked me these questions I grew more upset and concerned. How could I tell them when I didn't know myself? I'd seen a variety of registrars and a consultant who didn't know why I'd been referred to him. How was I to find out? A GP friend realised my problem. 'You do have a right to see the consultant' she informed me. 'Just ring up and insist that you see him.' So I did.

I had pinned a lot of hopes on that consultation and that someone would eventually give me a clear plan of what my future medical requirements would be. I was disappointed. Dr Fraser was a middle-aged man, quietly spoken. He apologised that we had not met before.

'What will be the follow-up procedure from now on?' I jumped in almost before he had finished, I was eager to know.

'Well, we'll just keep an eye on you.' Long pause.

'How often will the scans be then?'

'Oh, we won't scan you, we'll just keep an eye on you.'

What was he going to do, look for signs of tumour with his naked eye, or did he have X-ray vision?

'How will I know if it does come back?' I wanted to be sure that I gave myself every possible chance by catching it soon.

'You could have bleeding from somewhere you don't expect, or find strange lumps. I think really the best thing you can do is to try to forget that you have a sword hanging over your head and try to get on with your life' he finished with false empathy and smiled a forced smile.

He's obviously been on some communication skills training course and is trying to put it in to practice, I thought. It was blatantly not his style. How could he possibly know what it was like? It was very easy to say and hard to do.

I continued my questions, asking him about the long-term effects of the treatments.

'We don't really know', he smiled that awful smile again, he was probably just shy, 'because the drugs are so new. You do know that you could be infertile?'

I did. Was there any way of finding out? I needed to know the effects that the treatments had had on my body.

'Oh yes, in a few years time, once you're older and married we would be able to carry out some investigation.'

'Older and married', the same problem again. Separating patient's treatment from value judgements. Why did I have to be older than 26 or married to want children? Cancer affects people in such different ways. It could easily have encouraged me to want to leave such a mark on the world.

'Let's hope they've got it' he continued dolefully. 'You never can tell. Of course you've had all the treatment now, the chemo and everything, so there really wouldn't be much else I could do for you, except for clinical trials.'

A negative message to take away. I hardly felt better for that consultation.

My family was upset, they too had anticipated some answers, some direction. 'You need to know what is happening, catch it early if it is coming back. Go and see someone else' they counselled. But I had had enough of trailing round hospitals.

'I'm sure he knows his stuff otherwise he wouldn't be there' I argued. 'He's just an abysmal communicator.' The story was recounted to a family friend, an oncologist, who agreed.

'Oh he's very good at his job, but utterly hopeless with people' he told us, suggesting that I try someone else. 'Everyone says that about him.' At least it wasn't just me.

Surely people were an essential part of his job? Given my previous experiences of differing opinions, and advice regarding which doctors were desirable to see, I needed to establish faith in a doctor, for them to establish their credibility with me. A dearth of communication skills made this difficult to do. I was reassured to hear that his colleagues found him credible, respecting his technical knowledge and skills.

I was glad that things were progressing more smoothly as far as my psychological health was concerned. I had, Dr Withall explained, to see a psychiatrist for medical insurance purposes, who would then make a referral to a psychologist. I was quite intrigued to see how differently a psychiatrist would operate from a psychologist. Our discussion, if I can call it that, at his private rooms, involved me doing a lot of talking and him a lot of frantic scribbling, filling up pages of his A4 pad. It was a strange process for me. I was resurfacing and reiterating the issues that I had already dealt with, giving summarised versions of the outcomes. I knew that what I needed was to deal with the current concerns and pressures that were swimming around my head. I wanted to blurt these out, but they wouldn't make sense without the complicated background story I had embarked on. I had to provide a context before I dumped my bundle of present thought in to his lap.

In some respects I wanted to be a patient and let someone else tell me what I 'should' do but, having managed my own disease and treatment decisions throughout, I was used to having control. I felt sure that what I needed was continuing psychological support to deal with the issues that I was facing now that I was back in England. I was looking back on the previous year's events, and at the same time trying to look forward, rebuilding the future that had been shattered by my disease. I needed an objective listener to help me to juggle these two diametric perspectives, somebody outside of my family and friends, who could help me deal with cancer as a chronic illness, something that did not finish as soon as the treatment stopped. As I explained bluntly to Dr Lindsay, 'I don't want to be screwed up when I'm fifty about having had cancer in my twenties.'

Dr Lindsay agreed that a psychologist was a good option. I was uncomfortable taking antidepressants alone without any cognitive support, I had explained. My sister, also a psychologist, had been involved in some research at Oxford, investigating the combined use of cognitive and drug therapy. On her recommendation I was loath to use just one approach alone. Dr Lindsay also felt that a dual therapy would be effective, but managed to set my mind at rest about antidepressants. Radiation and cranial surgery, he informed me, could both cause depression through their physical effects, regardless of the psychological effects of the associated experiences. So it was like treating diabetes with insulin, depletion in the level of the neurochemical serotonin. A physical condition too, that sat more comfortably with me. I still felt that depression was a sign of my inability to cope with my situation and experiences and that I should be able to deal with it, get it together, particularly now that I was recuperating. Having a physical reason allowed me to be kinder to myself.

Dr Lindsay and I discussed my idea of writing a book.

'You may not want to go over the whole thing again' he warned me. 'Denial can sometimes be very effective.'

'I'm sure it can' I replied, 'after all, it is a highly evolved response. It obviously serves a very necessary purpose for human beings. It's just that I don't want to take what I see as the easy option. I don't want to think that I went through all of that for nothing, that nothing positive came out of it. I'm sure that a lot of doctors never get any feedback about how their patients feel. People probably either die or go into denial, not wanting to relive their painful experiences. I had no idea what cancer involved until I was suddenly thrown in to the middle of the cancer world. My only concept of cancer was that it killed, slowly and with considerable pain. I have a picture in my mind of the slides that a photographer friend had taken of his father's dead and emaciated body as a way of dealing with his own grief. I want to be able to explain to people what the treatment actually involves. How cancer affects your life. How you really feel.' I trailed off, not having fully formed the concept in my own mind.

'Yes' he mused, 'that could be really helpful, I mean if you could do it.' He told me about a book that his brother had recommended, written by a woman whose thesis had been on medical mistakes and had then, ironically, died due to a diagnostic error herself. 'It was powerful to read about her first hand experiences.'

CHAPTER 8

A panoramic view – the background picture

When Rachel wrote this final chapter, it was with the aim of identifying research to support her feelings about her experiences. She also wanted to summarise the wealth of research material, making it equally available to health professionals, cancer patients, and their relatives. Her intention was to finalise the chapter in collaboration with a medical professional: but sadly she ran out of time. We have taken the liberty of editing it, consulting with experts – the vast bulk of it, however, remains Rachel's work. We have then written an additional chapter, which follows, drawing out the main lessons as we see them.

My story is the tale of an individual, her thoughts, feelings and experiences recounted as they are logged in the archives of her memory. But how does it compare, in its twists and turns, to the experiences of others? The experiences of the numerous cancer patients and their relatives, of the GPs, oncologists and other health professionals working in the area? Cancer is frighteningly common. Current figures suggest that it touches one family in three. National newspapers carry articles weekly, proclaiming medical break-throughs or warning of new risk factors and concerns. Its nature and its prevalence beg a multitude of questions regarding the psychological aspects of both the treatment and management of cancer patients and their disease. As I charted my progress through the murky water of my disease and its treatment, and as I sat down to remember, to retell my story, a multitude of questions collected in my mind. Could the diagnosis have been handled more effectively? Did other patients feel upset and dissatisfied by clumsy consultation and ineffectual communication skills? Was I unusual in my desire for information and involvement in decision making? To what extent did other patients need or exercise control over their disease process? And from the other side, how did doctors feel about the training and support they were given in handling such difficult consultations? My questions went on, each experience I had had added a further layer of complexity, overlapping and enfolding each other like the petals of a tightly curled rose bud.

My questioning gathered pace, engulfing the issues of communication, control and decision making like a rolling snowball, and continuing on. There was so much more that I needed answering. What was the role of alternative and complementary therapies? Was I unusual to try them? Why did people seek them out? Could they work? I also queried the psychological aspects of cancer. Were personality and stress, oft mooted by the media to be contributors to developing the 'killer' disease, really relevant? How important was social support and quality of life? Was there a role for psychotherapy?

I myself had become convinced that the mind played an active and critical role in both the quality of an individual's existence, and also in their recovery. The psychological effects of the treatment process were, I believed, vitally important. My awareness of the role of communication and its impact was particularly heightened due to my background as an occupational psychologist. It so obviously had a key role in influencing the patient's frame of mind and ongoing adjustment. My questioning mind, combined with the desire to illustrate my subjective story with some objectivity, prompted me to begin my search, digging around among the rapidly growing research findings in the relevant literary allotment, psychosocial oncology, in a quest for understanding which would go some way to providing answers.

As is typical of research, the deeper I delved, the more conflicting viewpoints I unearthed. I have, however, attempted to provide a brief illumination of the current thinking and practice surrounding some of the area's key issues and concerns. I seek only to provide an overview, with references for further investigation and information, as the reader desires.

Alternative and complementary therapies

Complementary treatments are becoming more widely used and far more available. They encompass a wide range of approaches and philosophies, from acupuncture and Ayurveda, the eastern approaches, to homeopathy, herbalism, specific diets and crystal healing. With such a selection to choose from, the 'consumer' is rather like a child in a sweet shop, surrounded by jars of beautifully coloured sweets, but with all the labels removed. So what do people select and why?

Studies show that 25–45% of patients investigate avenues of complementary treatments.[1] They either use these in addition to orthodox treatments, or alone, if conventional treatments have failed, or are unacceptable to their spiritual or religious beliefs.[2] Alternatives are also pursued by those who are frustrated by the lack of information and certainty the conventional system has offered them. Primarily these patients are seeking a cure for their disease, a cure that cannot be guaranteed by conventional medicine. However, in addition to this curative search and the possible alleviation of the side effects of conventional treatments, complementary therapies can offer the patient something that is often sadly lacking in the conventional medical system, namely control. The typical traditional doctor–patient interaction consists of a significant imbalance of power. It is an involuntary relationship, which has been devastatingly thrust upon the patient, who is understandably afraid and vulnerable. The doctor holds all the cards, the specialist knowledge, the treatment technology.[1,2] In seeking alternative therapies the patient is often seeking to regain control, choice and independence. By respecting the patient's autonomy and exploration of complementary approaches, the doctor can also influence the patient's psychological adjustment and state of hopefulness. A further, broader, hypothesis for the appeal of such investigations has also been offered, suggesting that 'resorting to complementary medicine is perhaps an attempt to revert to traditional remedies, those of the origins and roots of humanity', in an intuitive quest for survival.[3]

Whatever the reason for an individual adopting an alternative approach, the existence of such an extensive framework of complementary medicine points to significant gaps in the conventional system. The obvious examples are the asymmetry of the doctor–patient relationship, and the lack of certainty of a cure. However, there is a broader issue, treatment of the whole person. In conventional medicine we treat 'bits' of a person. Their diseased lung, the nausea they experience as a side effect, their resulting anxiety. We do little to address the spiritual and psychological aspects of the individual within the world. This is not the case with some of the older, eastern approaches. The Chinese system ties up the physical symptoms with energy imbalance, which can be altered through the meridians (energy paths) of the body. It also links the interior of the body with the exterior and the cosmos. The patient's disease therefore becomes part of a far greater energy framework. Heading due south, the Indians practise an ancient medical system called Ayurveda, which translates as 'the science of life'. It also treats the whole individual by means of meditation, yoga, herbs, and diets tailored to the individual's body constituents. As with the ancient Greeks' theory of four body humours (phlegm, yellow bile, black bile and blood), disease is believed to come from imbalance. So these ancient systems treat disease as a result of some form of imbalance. This leads on to an additional role for a number of the alternative therapies. In our age of rational explanation, the aetiology of many tumours is still unexplained but, creatures of the 20th century, we need and demand explanations. Searching for answers leads us backwards, to the roots of ancient medicine, to help us explain the underlying reasons for the development of disease.

Certain 'alternatives' are in fact already being adopted in western hospitals, where relaxation and visualisation are techniques frequently employed with cancer patients. Whether or not treatments actually have an impact on disease outcome, they certainly play a significant role in the lives of many cancer patients. They can undoubtedly influence the quality of individuals' lives, if only by restoring control and hopefulness, or by addressing the side effects of conventional treatments. These factors alone are reason enough to regard alternative and complementary therapies as a beneficial adjunct to the conventional treatment of cancer.[4]

Communication

All of us can tell stories of visits to doctors, dentists or nurses, when we have left the consultation feeling dissatisfied, angry, or upset. Maybe we were not provided with the information that we expected, or we felt that our concerns had not been fully recognised or understood. Admittedly, this is sometimes to be expected; none of us can be perfect communicators a hundred per cent of the time. However, there are certain 'bone china' situations which are particularly fragile and sensitive, deserving and demanding more thoughtful and considered communication. The cancer diagnosis is a critical example.

Diagnosis

The diagnosis is one of the most difficult situations in which two individuals can find themselves. They have been thrown together in an involuntary relationship, in which they are occupying very unequal positions. The purpose for the discussion is vitally important and yet highly emotionally laden. Often there may have been little prior contact between the two, they may well, as it was in my case, be virtual strangers.[5,6] It is therefore no one's idea of the perfect situation in which to deliver or receive such devastating news. Bad news is difficult to give, even if one is required to do so on a regular basis, as well as to receive. I myself faced an obviously distressed doctor as my messenger of bad tidings. Doctors' fears surrounding the 'bad news' consultation are several fold. These include being blamed by the patient for the disease or outcome, or unleashing emotional reactions in the patient and expressing emotions themselves, not knowing all the answers and fear of the unknown and untaught. The situation also surfaces their own fears of illness and death. Although so blatantly sensitive and difficult for both parties, the diagnosis consultation is critical. It has even been mooted that 'The manner in which a physician discloses to a patient the diagnosis of cancer can, in itself, determine whether the patient will die or survive'.[7]

There are a number of differing guidelines for doctors on the theme of 'How to approach the diagnostic consultation'. These do, however, vary significantly in their recommendations.[8–11] When patients' views are sought it is evident that they too 'possess a plethora of opinions about how, where, and by whom cancer diagnoses are presented'.[12] What is clear is that there is no one 'set' way to conduct such an interview. The variation in research findings emphasises the need for interviews to be adapted to the individual, based on both the verbal and non-verbal cues that the patient provides.[13] These cues will be more easily picked up by those healthcare professionals who are 'natural communicators' than those who are unable to interpret, for example, shifts in body posture, or half-formed questions, or shy away from doing so through their own fear and discomfort.

There are several aspects of the diagnostic interaction which impact significantly on the overall level of satisfaction experienced by the patient. As the level of satisfaction is a known predictor of both compliance and psychological adjustment, and hence potentially of outcome, there are significant implications for the careful consideration of these factors in the case of each individual patient.[14–16]

Context

Patients consistently report that they would prefer the diagnosis to be done face-to-face, in privacy, by a doctor they know, but also with a specialist if the 'known' doctor cannot offer the appropriate expertise. They vary in whether they want to be accompanied by a friend or relative: some prefer to be told in total privacy, whereas others feel that they would benefit from the emotional support and extra pair of ears that a companion would bring to the consultation. They fail, however, quite unanimously, to welcome the inclusion of any semi-interested extras such as nurses or social workers.[12]

Preparation

The cancer diagnosis is a shocking and stunning blow, which lands surely and squarely between the eyes. Notwithstanding the nature of the disclosure, it is possible for this blow to be somewhat softened by employing skilful communication techniques. It can be easier for both if the doctor eases the individual into a discussion about their symptoms and the tests, therefore building up a background understanding of the patient and establishing what is already known, before delivering the devastating news.[17] In that way the doctor may lead the patient into recognising the severity and even the implications of their symptoms. The registrar who delivered my verdict was apparently wholly unaware that I did not know that my 'tumour' was in fact cancer.

Information

Doctors tend to believe that patients require information about the treatment of their disease. However this does not correspond with the requirements of patients, who feel that they need to know about the prognosis.[18,19] They also require emotional support and discussion of the treatment options available to them.[13,18] Patients are more satisfied with a consultation that addresses psychosocial issues and takes a counselling approach than they are with one that focuses purely on biomedical topics of conversation.[16] These are exactly the issues which are harder to deal with, requiring counselling and listening skills rather than reliance on hard facts. Research has shown that oncologists in fact significantly underestimate the level of distress that their patients are experiencing, and are therefore less likely to offer emotional support as they do not perceive the need.[20] It is understandably difficult to identify who might need the most support. This is neatly illustrated by the reasonable assumption that married women, with an assumed support network, will require less support than single women. However, they do in fact report the need for a significantly greater level, being unsure of who to turn to.[21] The requirements of the doctor's role will therefore vary significantly between patients and consultations.

How much to tell

This is a difficult question. The plethora of doctors I saw all had different ideas as to what I actually needed to know. The abiding tendency is for patients to want to have honest and meaningful information about their disease and a significant proportion feel that they would have liked more information than they actually received.[21] Doctors who try to protect their patients by sheltering them from painful disclosures may unwittingly be increasing their suspicion of a lethal outcome, and therefore increasing their anxiety.[22] That said, not all patients have similar information needs; there is a subgroup of patients who do not want to know anything about their disease. They may go into denial, convincing themselves that they do not have cancer and that this is not happening to them, or they may simply prefer to leave it all in the doctors' hands.[23]

The language and level of information required also vary considerably between patients. Some are very medically minded, whereas to others medical terminology can be very isolating and frightening. The terminology used in discussing cancer can affect patients' anxiety and vagueness and obscurity can affect long-term psychological adjustment.[24] My own lack of understanding of such words as 'oncology' and 'tumour', and their implications, meant that I was listening to a diagnosis that could just as well have been peppered with words of Swahili. Again this emphasises the importance of the tailoring of consultation styles to individual patients.

Questions and answers

It is difficult for patients who are in shock to remember what they have just been told, or to formulate the questions they want to ask. I think back to the questions that were tumbling around inside my head that I was unable to organise or articulate. Even if the questions are able to flow, patients can often experience considerable conflict in asking for the painful, personally relevant information.[2] Communication aids, including audio tapes of the consultation or a summary letter outlining the key aspects, have been shown to increase patient satisfaction. These are particularly useful for patients in relaying the information to friends and family, which can be difficult to remember or too painful to retell.[19] Patients may also need critical information to be repeated several times in order to take it on board. Even the most attentive students retain only 80% of what they're told in lectures, and they have not just been thrown into severe shock and confusion. Question prompt sheets can help patients to formulate some of the questions they may like to ask but are unable to put into words.[25] However, the doctor can also play an active role in helping the patient to articulate their questions and concerns by both questioning and silences, and by picking up on the cues by which the patient is reaching out for help.[26]

Hopefulness

There is evidence that profound hopelessness can have negative consequences for patients' prognosis and ongoing care. It is therefore logically considered that enhancing hopefulness, or positive thinking, can have a beneficial effect on cancer patients.[12] The diagnosis is the initial and critical encounter where the process of instilling hopefulness can begin. Patients can hope for a cure, however remote, and certainly for a remittance in the pain and discomfort they are experiencing as a result of the initial symptoms. Even in terminal cases it is possible for hope to be given, for example, that the individual's pain can be managed or that they can hope for a period of special time with their family. Some findings suggest that providing cancer patients with information that will assist them in coping with their problems can actually improve the overall clinical picture.[27,28] This has implications for the role of the doctor, suggesting that it is necessary 'to adopt an attitude of confident openness and to act as supportive and encouraging coaches rather than acting as detached clinicians or consoling care takers'.[12] It is certainly easier to run a race with constant and positive encouragement than with someone who is only interested in ensuring that the hurdles are in the appropriate places and the start to finish time in relation to the national average.

This is not to say, however, that health professionals should be encouraged to give their patients false hope of survival. For false hope can be equally as harmful to patients' psychological adjustment

and threaten feelings of trust between doctor and patient. It is important to remember that hope does not have to be solely based on cure,
but can also derive from expectation of quality of life and effective
pain management.

Ongoing communication

Patients report an ongoing need for information and, in a large
proportion of cases, for participation in decision making. Patients who
are active in decision making have been found to be more satisfied
with their treatment and more psychologically well-adjusted than
those who are passive. However, it cannot be assumed that patients
want to take on full responsibility for decision making and can be
presented with the sum total of clinical information and asked to make
a choice. The majority prefer the doctor to adopt the role of major
decision maker, but want to be an informed participant, exercising a
degree of psychological autonomy.[29,30] For the doctor to play this role
effectively they need to have a clear understanding of the patient's key
decision-making criteria, which may significantly differ from their
own. I know one of my doctors was particularly concerned about the
cosmetic effects of surgery, believing that it would be very mutilating.
I myself was far more concerned with achieving a cure. For the
patients, their participation, if desired, serves to reduce fears of over-
dependence on the doctor and can also lead to new learning and activities, and personal growth. Patients' needs for information may
change over the period of the disease, as the shock of diagnosis wears
off, or as the disease responds, develops or recurs. The emotional
support that a patient needs may also vary through the course of their
illness.[31] Families can be driven apart by the cancer diagnosis and the
stigma of cancer can lead to significant shifts and changes in the
individual's pre-cancer support network.[32,33] As the many influences
on the patient are not static, so the doctor–patient relationship
becomes, by necessity, a dynamic and ever-changing entity.

Doctor training

Patients most definitely view communication as a facet of medical
competence, yet many doctors do not receive the appropriate
ongoing training to effectively handle the complex and varied situations that are engendered by the cancer consultation.[14] They get

little feedback from their patients, as patients are often reluctant to criticise their doctors due to their dependence on them for medical treatment.[34,35] Rather like employees uncomfortable at the idea of giving open and honest feedback to a boss whom their job depends on. They themselves admit that they need further training in skills which allow them to accurately assess their patients' problems, and to counsel their patients and relatives effectively.[20] Training itself however is not enough. These doctors need to work within a system which overtly values interpersonal and communication skills, and has a reward system that recognises their worth. As research findings necessitate a broadening of the competencies demanded of the medical professionals, the system too must change to encompass and reinforce these requirements (*see* Chapter 9).

Quality of life

Cancer is no longer, due to advances in medical treatment, the kiss of death. Far more often it is now regarded as a chronic disease that the patient will live and survive with for many years. The ongoing quality of life of cancer patients has therefore become a more prominent concern, both for patients themselves, their relatives and those who are treating such patients. Cancer treatments can be very aggressive and comprehensive in their impact on patients' lives, affecting the physical, emotional and social aspects of their existence. It can be difficult to determine which of these treatments is worst, each has its own characteristic marks. Chemotherapy can produce side effects such as nausea and vomiting, hair loss, anxiety and digestive problems; radiotherapy can lead to symptoms including depression, anxiety, skin problems and asthenia; and surgery too can be mutilating and disfiguring. Decisions regarding treatment options therefore necessarily need to evaluate and balance the chances of survival with the subsequent quality of life left to the patient. So what is 'quality of life'?

A recent study suggested that there are four major aspects of the quality of a cancer patient's life – physical, psychological, support and existential.[36] The physical aspects are easy to identify: the physical side effects of treatments (e.g. hair loss, vomiting) and their permanent effects (e.g. amputation), along with the effects of the disease (e.g. pain, lumps or bleeding), are obviously visible, and can tend to be the major focus of a doctor's evaluation of a patient's quality of life. Studies have shown that doctors attribute far greater significance to physical factors than do patients. Patients, for example, do not prefer the more conservative approach of radio-therapy following chemotherapy for a sarcoma of the leg, over amputation, as might be expected. I myself preferred the more aggressive surgery option to the less disfiguring but potentially less effective radiotherapy alone.

The other three aspects are less visible. Support itself is multifaceted and discussed further under 'social support'. Psychological factors are also difficult to untangle and identify. The major disturbances of depression and anxiety have been outlined in the afore-named section. There are however other psychological issues that warrant discussion. A number of studies have examined patients' coping responses and their results suggest that patients whose coping response to their diagnosis is one of a 'fighting' approach have a longer duration of survival than those who respond in a passive, helpless way. It has also been suggested, equivocally, that denial can be related to good prognosis.[37] Another important issue for cancer patients, which has both psychological and physical origins, is that of sexual function. Although some of the physiological changes relating to cancer treatments can lead to sexual dysfunction, through pain, fatigue and hormonal changes, there is also a significant psychological component at play. Patients can often feel undesirable and devalued, experiencing low self-esteem and the fear of rejection.[3] Changes in body image and feminine identity have frequently been found to lead to sexual problems in women who have had mastectomies. Sexual problems are not simply unique to women or breast cancer patients. A large number of cancer patients report that the disease had an impact on their sexual activity at a time when they probably most needed the warmth, physical contact and relaxation that a sexual relationship could offer them. The issues of sexual dysfunction and also infertility, which often result from cancer treatments, can be difficult for both patients and doctors to discuss. However, a satisfying sex life contributes significantly to an individual's identity and self-esteem and thus is an important component in their overall quality of life.

The existential component of quality of life is defined as 'concerns regarding death (existential obliteration), freedom (the absence of external structure), isolation (the final unbridgeable gap separating self from all else), and the question of meaning (the dilemma of meaning-seeking creatures who recognise the possibility of a cosmos without meaning)'. This definition in itself demonstrates that the quality of life of cancer patients contains components that may be far less significant to those who are not facing a life threatening illness.

These are questions that can be regarded as more of a spiritual and philosophical nature, and understandably not within the realm in which any health professional would seek to offer unequivocal answers and advice. It does however raise questions that patients may seek to explore and discuss, whether it be with a doctor, minister, yoga teacher or partner. Recognition of and support in contemplation of these issues can assist an individual in the journey of their own personal development, thoughts and understanding.

In addition to the concept of considering the quality of a patient's existence, whether it be ten years or ten days, there is also the possibility that quality of life may have an impact on prognosis. Studies involving patients with melanoma and lymphoma[38] and breast cancer[39] have suggested that psychosocial intervention with the objective of enhancing participants' quality of life can lead to increased length of survival. It is difficult, however, due to the complexity of both situations and individuals, to identify which aspects of the intervention are most significant. For example, social support, problem solving or information may all play a role to a greater or lesser extent. In addition, cancer encompasses a wide variety of disease types, and it is hard to determine for which tumour and personality types such interventions could play a role.

Social support

Cancer to me, at the time of my diagnosis, was a disease that was closely associated with pain and death. Investigations examining the stigma of cancer have found that a significant proportion of people do believe that cancer is a death sentence and, in addition in some cases, that cancer is contagious.[40] Being in the presence of an individual with cancer can itself be unsettling as a reminder of one's own mortality. These social attitudes, combined with the discomfort of not knowing what to say or how to help, can lead to physical, social or psychological withdrawal, both from the patient's friends and relatives, or from the patients themselves. The nature of cancer, its treatments and their side effects can also lead to physical restrictions on the patient's social interactions. Someone suffering from nausea and hair loss is unlikely to be out playing tennis every day, or to be the life and soul of the party.

Social support is important to nearly all human beings as we progress through the undulating landscape of our lives. Evidence from the studies of bereavement and social relationships clearly demonstrates that a link between social ties could be of particular importance. There have, however, been equivocal and conflicting results from studies investigating these effects in cancer patients. In a study of breast cancer and melanoma patients, no association was found between social support and time to relapse.[41,42] In a group of patients with metastatic breast cancer, interventions involving weekly sessions focusing on coping mechanisms, feelings and self-hypnosis were found to increase survival rates; however this may not be purely attributable to the emotional support provided by such groups.[39] The evidence as to whether social connections are related to death from cancer is therefore a rather mixed bag.

There is, however, sufficient evidence to suggest that social support is related to physical and mental health and can affect an individual's quality of life.[43–5] Social support can be given in several ways: informational support, which can assist in problem solving and decision making; instrumental support, providing assistance with tasks such as transport or finance, that may actually get the treatment process moving smoothly and quickly; and emotional support which can have a considerable effect on distress, self-esteem and sense of control. The mechanisms by which these factors could play a role are several: by increasing the individual's coping mechanisms and hopefulness, through some psychoneuroimmunological mechanism, or by influencing 'lifestyle factors' which may influence the development, diagnosis and treatment of cancer. As yet, the precise role these factors play in the prevention and development of specific diseases is unclear; suffice it to say that currently there does appear to be some association whose shape and form are as yet undetermined.

Depression and anxiety

Psychological disturbances are common in cancer patients, throughout and after their formal treatment regime. Particular points where distress is likely to be the most acute have been clearly identified as diagnosis, treatment, advanced disease and recurrence.[46] Although such distress is to be expected, these symptoms are frequently severe enough to require pharmacological or psychological interventions.

The adjustment disorders of anxiety and depression are often found in cancer patients. However, diagnosis is not always simple and straightforward so symptoms often go unrecognised and untreated. Between 23% and 56% of patients are reported to suffer from depression. By the nature of the beast, depression can be difficult to diagnose in cancer patients. The depressive symptoms that cancer patients experience could easily be the result of the disease and its treatments, making it hard to determine whether the patient's depressive state has an emotional origin, or whether its roots are organic. For example, sleep disturbances and loss of appetite could result from chemotherapy treatment as well as from depression. The problem of diagnosis is further compounded by the psychiatric diagnostic criteria, which were not designed for use in patients with chronic illnesses, where individuals are unaware of and unprepared for the complex process of their treatment, and are suffering from a chronic illness, throughout which levels of distress can fluctuate significantly. Suggested symptomatic indicators in cancer patients have included self-concept, early morning waking, the ability to experience pleasure, diurnal variation in mood and views about the future.[47] The emphasis on on-going monitoring and identification lies heavily at the doctor's door. Depressed patients can characteristically fail to believe that anyone can help them, may just accept the symptoms as part of their illness or not want to waste precious time in a short consultation discussing psychological issues, so are often unlikely to ask for help.[48] Anxiety is also common among cancer patients, and somewhat easier to identify than depression. Patients are understandably afraid of pain and death, of losing control, abandonment, changes in body image and the recurrence of their disease. Tests, such as a bone marrow biopsy, and alienating treatments, including chemo and radiotherapies, can also provoke extreme levels of anxiety. Patients may appear to be on edge, and display variations in mood from which they cannot be distracted. They may also suffer from panic attacks, irritability, sweating, tremor and nausea, and initially experience insomnia. Again, some of these symptoms may be confused with the effects of the tumour or its treatments.

The identification and treatment of these psychological disturbances are imperative. They can have a profound effect on the individual's quality of life and affect their adherence to the treatment and their ability to make decisions, which could ultimately impact on their chance of survival.[49] Unfortunately oncologists often fail to detect not only general distress but also the psychological disorders that their patients are experiencing. They have been found to significantly under-rate their patients' distress, and themselves admit that they require training in psychological assessment.[20] This could also reflect the discomfort associated with probing that could let down the flood gates to a tidal emotional response. Those doctors who were most effective in identifying distress were those who allowed patients to express their concerns and picked up on the non-verbal (e.g. postural, movement) and verbal cues from their patients.[50]

So, in line with Galen's melancholic women, is depression itself a predisposing risk factor to developing cancer? The research suggests that it is not, concluding that the evidence is 'not consistent with a strong link between depressive symptoms and cancer',[51] although major segments of depression such as helplessness and depressed mood are associated with poor prognosis, supporting the idea that some people simply decide to give up on life or, in terms of more eastern philosophies, shut off from their life force.[52,53]

Intervention and psychotherapy

A number of different intervention approaches have been adopted to address the problems related to cancer and its treatments. This array has included individual psychotherapy, group therapy, general behaviour therapies tailored for use with cancer patients and psychopharmacology. So what roles do these interventions play? Do they simply deal with the psychosocial effects of cancer or can they actually have an effect on prognosis?

Psychotherapy has generally been employed to help the individual to manage the trauma that they experience at the diagnosis, and to come to terms with its implications for personal meaning.[54] As the disease process progresses it also plays a role in assisting patients in coping with their disease and maintaining as reasonable a quality of life as circumstances permit.[55] The benefits of such an approach have been found to include a reduction in levels of distress and a better resolution of problems in addition to lower levels of depression, anxiety and hostility, coupled with an increased likelihood of a return to previous employment.[56,57] For certain patients undergoing particular medical protocols such as radiotherapy, psychotherapy has been found to be effective in the reduction of both emotional stress and physical symptoms.[58] It has also been used extensively with terminally ill patients, aiding them in a realistic coping with their disease and coming to terms with approaching death.[59]

Group therapies have also been popular. The objectives of such therapies are multifold. They aim to enable support, sharing of feelings, the development of coping skills, the gathering of information and education and the consideration of existential issues.[60]

Group therapy can include the family, friends and carers of cancer patients, and may therefore be more acceptable to individuals who are uncomfortable with the idea of individual therapy. The most commonly used approach to group therapy is that of support, which has been found to reduce both emotional distress and psychosocial problems.[61] However, a comparison of supportive groups with coping skills instruction discovered that the facilitation of coping in the patients had a far greater impact, resulting in significant improvements in effect, satisfaction with lifestyle activities, cognitive distress, communication and coping with medical procedures.[62] The variety of group therapies employed and the dynamic context in which the cancer patient sits make it difficult to determine the precise mechanism and magnitude of these frequently reported effects.

Behaviour therapies and cognitive behaviour therapies are techniques that have been widely used for general purposes and have been adapted for use with cancer patients. Therapies such as systematic desensitisation and progressive muscle relaxation, in conjunction with guided imagery, have been used to treat specific symptoms, including nausea, vomiting and emotional distress resulting from chemotherapy.[63,64] Behaviour therapy has also been employed to address some of the adjustment disorders experienced by cancer patients, particularly anxiety and depression and to address issues of self-esteem.[65,66] One example of a behavioural approach is adjuvant psychological therapy (APT).[67] It is based on the view that the interpretations and evaluations which the patient assigns to their illness determine the emotional distress that they experience. It has two principal objectives – to reduce anxiety, depression and other psychiatric symptoms, and to improve mental adjustment to cancer by inducing a positive fighting spirit. It is problem solving oriented and focuses on restructuring the patient's thoughts, encouraging the development of new and effective coping strategies. It has been shown, in specific studies, to be successful in achieving its objectives.[68]

Antidepressants and anxiolytic drugs are frequently used to treat depression and anxiety in cancer patients. Although an effective short term treatment and critical in treating purely physical depression, there is clearly an additional role for cognitive and behavioural therapies. This is supported by findings that a combination of the two approaches has been more effective than a pharmacological approach alone in the treatment of breast cancer patients.[63] Combination treatments were also found to have a longer lasting effect than antidepressants alone.[69]

The variety of interventions discussed can obviously have a significant impact on the cancer patient's quality of life. But can they prolong survival? The researchers in this area stand divided. There are several studies which have found that psychosocial intervention[64] including behaviour therapy[70] and supportive group therapy[39] have lead to longer survival times. However, other findings have failed to support such conclusions.[42] There have also been some suggestions that specific types of psychological intervention may actually lead to a poorer prognosis.[71,72] So, the crystal ball contains nothing but swirling mists. However, the balance of findings led one researcher to sum up the current state of thinking by the conclusion that 'psychological intervention, in the form of counselling or supportive psychotherapy, might provide some survival advantage but, more importantly, may improve quality of survival'.[73]

CHAPTER 9

The messages for health professionals

John Hasler and David Pendleton

Introduction

Rachel has written an evocative and moving account of her final illness. In this she has succeeded in describing a range of feelings, including frustration, sadness, despair and humour. At the same time she has managed to combine this with an understanding of the communication between her and the professionals, often seeing the problems from the professionals' point of view, even on the occasions when she felt let down and demoralised.

We recognise that this is one side of the picture and that memories and recollection of events often do not reveal the true state of affairs – there are always two sides to a story. But our experience tells us that her account of events is by no means unusual. One of us is a doctor, who worked in general practice and medical education for many years and is only too conscious of his own failings in the past. The other is a psychologist with a particular interest in doctor–patient communication, with real insights into the challenge faced by doctors every day of the week, and sympathy with the predicaments in which those doctors find themselves. For Rachel's sake we try here to draw out the messages for those involved in the care of patients, not just patients with cancer but all those who seek help through their consultations.

Consulting effectively

Rachel's story describes a journey from life to death. It is powerful, painful and disturbing. On her way, Rachel passes first from person to patient. For Rachel, this seems to have been one of the more disturbing transitions. Rachel was a psychologist and management consultant. She was used to weighing evidence and coming to conclusions. She often dealt with powerful people in senior positions. She was also fit and healthy for most of her life. Yet, once she became a patient, she was treated by some of her carers in a way that seemed to deny her identity, education and experience.

Most readers respond emotionally to Rachel's story. We did, and we joined in the chorus of 'How could they?' and 'How dare they?' Yet the best response any of us could make is to learn from it, and not look to blame or criticise. Rachel's carers varied considerably. Some understood her need for information and certainty and did their best to meet it. Others responded to her vulnerability and tried to protect her as best they could. A few seemed not to respond to her needs at all, but who knows what was happening in their lives at the time.

Medical care is very hard to practise well. It requires a delicate and difficult blend of science and art, discipline and flexibility, dispassionate evaluation of evidence and deep caring humanity. Some practitioners insulate themselves from the tragedy and pain by moving entirely towards the scientific and the dispassionate. In so doing, they run the risk of denying their own and their patient's humanity and of no longer caring. Others become overwhelmed by their feelings and run the risk of not being able to help their patients at all. Those of us who are involved in training, coaching and managing carers do well to steer them between these rocks at either side of their path.

To learn from Rachel's experience, we have to understand what makes all medical care effective. We need a model of effective consulting and a means of helping doctors, nurses and other professionals to practise in this way.

Most consultations are relatively easy to locate on a continuum that runs from doctor-centred to patient-centred. Doctor-centred consultations are dominated by the medical agenda in which the role of the patient is to answer questions, not ask them. Doctor-centred consultations focus on the disease rather than the person, they inform rather than involve and they expect patients to do as they are told. They originate from a view of the doctor as a technical specialist: an expert in scientific medicine.

Patient-centred consultations are dominated by the patient's agenda. They treat the whole person rather than the disease, they involve patients in the diagnostic process as well as the choice of treatments, and they share uncertainty with patients. They are also much more difficult to do well than are doctor-centred consultations since they require the careful balancing of many conflicting factors.

The balance of evidence strongly suggests that patient-centred consultations are more effective in terms of outcomes achieved: short term, medium term and longer term. In the short term, patients are more satisfied when they are given more information. In the medium term, patients follow treatment plans more closely when they are involved in the decision making. In the longer term, patients tend to show greater improvements in their health when they are given more control of the consultation process and more say in the decisions made.[74,75]

The patient-centred style takes account of the patient's perspective: her ideas about health and the problem presented, her concerns about the problem and its treatment, and her expectations of the doctor. The patient-centred style also recognises that patients regularly ask themselves, and would like to ask the doctor, five questions:

- What could be wrong?
- Why has it happened?
- Why to me?
- Why now?
- What will happen now?

All consultations need to deal with these issues. Rachel's experience would have been very different if *all* her carers had held these questions in their minds and attempted to deal with them.

The patient-centred style also involves patients in all aspects of their care. Patient-centred doctors make their diagnoses together with their patients and ensure that patients understand the evidence they have taken into account. They also come to treatment decisions with patients, allowing them to weigh the options and to fashion a treatment plan that will work for them, taking account of their needs and lifestyle.

Pendleton *et al.* have described the tasks of patient-centred consulting and practical ways in which these tasks may be achieved.[76] They have also described how these tasks may be both taught and learned. The tasks are:

Understand the problem

Understand the patient. Patients come with 'problems' rather than diseases and the professional's task is to understand these problems, so that management can be directed whenever possible at the causes rather than just the effects. This also includes understanding the patient's illness experience. This comprises both the *effects* that the problems may be having on the patient's life, as well as the sense that the patient is making of the whole experience. Patients always seek to make some sense of their experience, and it is this drive that contributes to the patient's perspective. This is a complex task to achieve in its entirety, and the strategies and skills required to understand the problem's nature and history and its aetiology are of a different order from those required to explore the patient's perspective.

Illnesses also have meanings and implications for patients that can generate *concerns*. Establishing what these are enables the doctor to offer appropriate reassurance, empathy, or support. There is good evidence that addressing patients' concerns is also therapeutic.

Most consultations include some decisions about investigations, treatment and management. Patients will sometimes attend with specific *expectations* about these matters. It is wise to deal with these expectations explicitly. Patients will also vary in the extent to which they expect to be informed and involved in decisions about their care. It would seem self-evident that understanding why the patient has really come is the essential first task in any consultation, and indeed Byrne and Long found that failure to do so was the commonest cause of dysfunctional consultations.[77] The crucial point about agendas is that they are often concealed because of fear, embarrassment or uncertainty.

Share understanding

Most patients want to be told about their problem and its management in ways that they can remember and understand. Their satisfaction with the consultation is substantially influenced by the amount of information they are given. Additionally, reduction of uncertainty is in itself therapeutic. They need to be informed in order to enable them to manage the problem themselves more effectively. Patients cannot participate in shared decision making about treatment unless they understand the options and their implications.

There will be some consultations in which explanations are required about the risks and benefits of treatment. This raises the issue about how such explanations are framed. Words may have meanings that are not clearly understood, and medical usage may be somewhat different from common use. Similarly, percentages or other figures may be interpreted in different ways. For example, patients are more likely to take a treatment if told that it will reduce their risk of another heart attack by a third than if they are told that it reduces their risk from 12% to 8%.

Most consultations involve uncertainty and we would argue that part of the task is to help patients understand and tolerate it rather than seek to protect them from it. We believe the underlying ethos must be honesty but this will often mean acknowledging the frailties of medical predictions and prognostications. The medical profession has not done anyone any favours in the past by pretending that diagnosis is always possible, that screening will detect all abnormalities, and that treatments are risk free.

Achieving a shared understanding is not the same as explaining to the patient. An explanation is a one-way process, from doctor to patient, a sharing of understanding is a two-way process and cannot occur unless the patient's perspective has been elicited in the first phase.

Doctors sharing understanding are also formulating management plans whilst talking and listening. The act of sharing understanding is intended to clarify, modify and tailor the subsequent decision, thus making it more appropriate. Much of the effective sharing will be in the emotional realm, of wants, needs, fears and irrational beliefs. It is also important to realise that patients' expectations of medicine's capacity to deliver diagnosis and cure almost always outstrip the reality. This is a true understanding and not one that some patients wish to acknowledge.

Share decisions and responsibility. In the majority of consultations decisions are made either explicitly or implicitly about management, and choices are made between options ranging from doing nothing to self-care, prescription or further investigations or procedures. The headline issue is whether these decisions are made by the doctor, the patient or the two of them together. The underlying issue is *how* the decisions are made.

The classic decision making process is to define the problem, define the options, consider the advantages and disadvantages of each option, and then decide. In a medical decision, the options have potential benefits and risks, with differing probabilities. Different patients will have different views according to their life stages. They may need help and time to consider the implications of the options for them before the decision is made. Doctors can not only provide information but also offer their opinion, and many patients prefer them to do so. Sharing the decision is about sharing information and opinions, and helping patients understand and consider the options, in a balanced way. At best, the doctor can state the probabilities but only the patient can weight them appropriately.

For the patient to participate in major decisions of the sort Rachel had, more time may be required than is available in a single consultation. In this circumstance, offering patients time to consider and indicating other sources of information is an important ingredient in shared decision making.

Maintain the relationship

The essential point about this task is that it defines a desirable doctor–patient relationship in terms of its effectiveness rather than any preconceived ideas of correctness. According to this definition, an effective relationship is one in which patients are able to state their ideas and concerns, in which sharing of information and decisions take place, and one in which a partnership between the patient and the doctor is built.

A relationship can also be assessed in terms of its therapeutic effectiveness. As well as achieving the tasks, the extent to which a doctor displays warmth, genuineness and unconditional positive regard for their patients also determines an effective therapeutic relationship. There is, however, more to the relationship that has implications for the doctor than warmth and regard, there are also responsibilities. The place of trust is also probably crucial to outcome.

One of the biggest threats to the doctor–patient relationship is the rise of defensive patterns in the consultation. Salinsky and Sackin have elucidated this area in their book *What Are You Feeling, Doctor?*[78] They point out several defensive strategies used frequently by doctors to avoid emotional involvement. These include retreating totally into clinical medicine, always steering the conversation to the organic and so safely into tests, referrals and prescriptions.

There is also a danger that the relationship may become too cosy and is preserved at all costs. It may be to help doctors complete the tasks more effectively that they will need training in self-awareness, a greater recognition of the forces that create defensive patterns of consulting and greater help with emotional understanding. The effective relationship required to facilitate the tasks is not emotionally neutral. It carries emotional risk and requires real involvement with another human being in the form of genuine enthusiasm and true caring.

All this can seem like a tall order, but it is what professionals need to aim for.

Co-ordinating several specialities

There is potential enough for things to go amiss when just one doctor or nurse is involved. But when several are involved the possible difficulties begin to multiply. In the first place there is the question of how far doctors within one team have kept each other informed – not an easy matter when the pressures of work and move to shift systems provide less opportunity. Rachel's description of the registrar assuming that she knew the nature of her diagnosis illustrates this point vividly. And later – 'I just don't know what to do. I keep getting different answers and I don't know who is right, I don't know what to do.'

The nature of cancer treatment is that it is likely to involve more than one speciality – surgeons, sometimes from more than one speciality as in Rachel's case; oncologists; pathologists; radiologists; radiotherapists, and so on. On top of that there are all the other professionals – nurses; radiographers; physiotherapists; to name but three. Any psychologist will tell you that the number of possible communication channels and the scope for information not being shared by all the key people are legion. At every stage of the diagnosis and treatment, patients will ask questions of a range of people with whom they come into contact. And if that isn't bad enough, all this takes place in a highly charged atmosphere of human mortality. In these situations words are often misheard or not heard at all.

Communication issues between teams and professionals are not confined to malignant disease. There are many other chronic and acute conditions where more than one specialist team is involved and often where more than one professional has a hand in treatment.

Clearly there are many situations where communication and co-ordination work well and the frequency of these should not be underestimated. But if patients are confused, to whom should they turn? In Britain the logical answer will often be the patient's general practitioner. In theory GPs receive all the communications about each individual patient and there are good arguments for them adopting the role of interpreter. They often have a long-standing relationship with the patient, which involves not simply the details of their medical history but how these patients react to information, what kind of language it should be conveyed in, and their resilience to stress and bad news. They know which patients they can joke with and those with whom they would never dare to do so. They know how strong their patients' views are and how much control they like to exert in their dealings with health professionals. All GPs have experience of acting as interpreter after a specialist consultation and obtaining further information on the patient's behalf. If co-ordination is needed and it is not occurring, it seems to us that the GP should step in.

However, when it comes to cancer, particularly the treatment and monitoring stages, this may be easier said than done, nor is it always appropriate. The frequency of attendances involved with radiotherapy or chemotherapy often means that the patient's relationship with their GP is temporarily interrupted as the patient transfers their main ongoing relationship to the specialist concerned. Furthermore, the GP is often unaware of the latest twist in the saga or lacks the latest information from the hospital. In Rachel's case, when the diagnosis was revealed she grabbed the doctor with whom she felt she could talk most easily. So, we'd say, if you are a GP with a patient involved with numerous specialists, check it out and ask the patient how they are getting on and if they have someone who is co-ordinating the orchestra.

Second opinions and alternative therapies

There will be times when the patient or the doctor considers a second opinion or some form of alternative therapy. How should these questions be best handled? For the doctor, such a request by a patient implies that somehow the original doctors did not know what they were doing. And in the process, there is an implication that maybe this applies to the medical profession as a whole. A wise doctor recognises that his colleagues, like himself, are human, and responds appropriately. One of us can recall a situation of a diagnosis of malignancy which turned out to be benign, and another situation where a patient, whose condition was considered terminal, was given five further years of good quality life by a different hospital. Equally, there will be times when the patient has to be dissuaded from shopping around, in the hope that cure is possible when it is not. Sometimes it is the doctor himself who suggests a second opinion or alternative therapy, balancing a possible benefit against raising false hopes. All of these need handling with sensitivity and judgement.

The need for the patient to have control

It is sometimes difficult for doctors to appreciate the feelings of loss of control felt by many patients when they become ill or medicalised. We are used to making our own decisions about what we will do, when we will do it, and generally taking charge of our lives. But patients suddenly find that they are no longer masters of their fate, that others are making decisions for them, or worse still that their own bodies have got out of control, interfering with their ability to do everything they want.

We have seen that it is important for doctors to understand these feelings and frustration and to involve patients, as far as possible, in their own decisions about treatment and management. One can appreciate Rachel's frustration in the sudden shift from autonomy in her early days in Sydney to becoming a dependent creature at the mercy of others and her cancer.

Perhaps all doctors would benefit from being patients early in their careers. But if that is not possible – and we would not want to wish illness on anyone, doctor or not – what else can the doctors do to enable them to understand their patients' feelings? There is now a considerable amount of teaching around consultations, especially for future general practitioners. The use of videotape to record, observe and analyse consultations has been in widespread use for many years whilst methods of assessing consultations have been developed to help doctors understand what is happening. However, in our experience, most of the learning and teaching takes place with only doctors present. On the rare occasions when the patient has been invited in to discuss the consultation as well, the learning experience for the doctors is often powerful. On occasions, patients also used to join more general group discussions of young doctors – indeed one of us used to do this regularly on day release courses for GP registrars. On these occasions the patients' comments are considerably more powerful than points the teacher can presume to make.

Taking responsibility

It's very easy and entirely logical, when things go wrong due to administrative problems elsewhere in the system, for health professionals to wash their hands of these problems, since after all they are faults that have nothing to do with them. Moreover, the busier health professionals and their supporting staff become, the more likely it is that administrative arrangements will come adrift.

We need to remember that it is often difficult enough for those who work in the system to sort out why appointments have gone astray, why scans get postponed for 24 hours or why the hospital records can't be found (how often does that happen?). Rachel again – 'We wandered about the ward looking for assistance, eventually tracking down an absent minded registrar.' If it's difficult for the staff, how much more difficult is it for the patient, especially when they are ill, demoralised, or confused? So even when it is not the direct concern of the person in the firing line, that person at that moment represents the health system and needs to take responsibility for doing what they can to sort things out. Attempting to explain to the patient the reasons for the mistake is not particularly helpful, what the patient wants is to have it sorted out. We have all had the frustrating experience of trying to get helpful answers on the phone, only to be passed from one person to another while Vivaldi's *Four Seasons* tinkles in our ear, and an electronic voice says 'Your call is important to us'.

Conclusions

In our experience, whenever we have introduced the patient's voice into learning sessions for health professionals, these sessions have been powerful and relevant experiences. And so, we believe, has Rachel's voice, coming to us from the pages she penned in her final years.

The future for healthcare is an increasing partnership between patient and professional. Those of us who have experienced or witnessed consultations where that partnership has started to become alive have been struck by the increased satisfaction it brings to both parties. We have seen that the evidence supports a greater involvement in decision making by the patient, and the need to understand the patient's ideas, concerns and expectations. And, in the end, we are all patients.

Rachel's story could have been different. It could have been a story of involvement and sharing but she would still, nevertheless, have had to face a great deal of uncertainty and pain. Nor would her story have had a happier ending, just a different process in which the person would never have had to be subsumed by the patient.

CHAPTER 11

Epilogue

Naomi Jefferies

The epilogue Rachel penned in December 1996 read simply '???????'

She ended her narrative of 'orienteering oncology' still fiercely clinging to the belief that through sheer strength and will she would successfully navigate her way through the not just rocky, but mountainous, terrain of her life. Yet, her struggle was far from over.

In July 1996 she had spent the gruelling 25-hour flight from Sydney to Heathrow, full of sleeping tablets and well tended by the Quantas flight crew who were concerned by the appearance of her swollen, scarred face and tufty hair. So strong was her need for the comfort and security of home and the support of long-standing friends and family that she was keen not to delay her trip a minute longer than was necessary. She had initially come back for a holiday, to stay with our mother and to recuperate from the major surgery she had had shortly before leaving Sydney. However, once home she began to allow herself to realise the enormity of what had happened to her and to question her decision to return to Australia where she was in the process of applying for residency. Luckily Nick was still over in Sydney 'doing Oz' (a slightly more costly experience as he was now minus the free hospital meals). He arranged for her belongings to be shipped home, and for her little kitten, Molly, to be airlifted to friends with a farm out in the New South Wales countryside. No expense spared for this important little feline friend.

Her early few months back in England were mixed – with the pleasure of catching up with old friends and exploring old haunts, and the fear of the recurrence of the cancer. In the autumn Rachel started work back at the Coopers and Lybrand London office, joined a local health club and rented a small house in Putney with her great university friend Rik. Despite the semblance of a return to normality, the nagging doubt remained; how would she know if the tumour returned? Would she be able to catch it in time? And what would she do if it did come back?

Following a brief period of respite, the familiar symptoms of nasal congestion, sinus pains and incredible tiredness began to return. This time, however, her body was not as strong and healthy as the athletic body it had been only a year before. Her once straight hair was just starting to grow into lush, dark, 'chemo curls' when she started her rounds of consulting rooms once again.

I cannot even begin to mirror the depths of Rachel's writing or to give such a vivid and moving account of her following experiences. However, my description of her next, and last, two years can help to complete the picture. The return of Rachel's cancer was confirmed in the early summer of 1997. One Sunday she arrived for a family lunch at our aunt Morwenna's house. It was a beautiful sunny morning, a day filled with the promise of summer barbecues and badminton in the garden. She parked her car in the drive and walked up to the house. The minute we saw her in the drive we knew that it was back. Although beautifully dressed, she looked grey and something in her eyes confirmed her second sense that something was wrong. A consultation with Dr Fraser the next week confirmed these fears; the tumour in her sinus was sizeable, although he suggested it was possibly treatable by further surgery and chemotherapy.

Her summer months, leading into autumn, were peppered with stays in one of the London hospitals to receive chemotherapy. One of the unfortunate side effects of chemotherapy is to lower the white blood cell count significantly, thus reducing the person's immunity. At the times when Rachel's white cell count was particularly low she was moved into an isolation room, where visitors and the medical team alike were required to wear white plastic aprons and 'hibiscrub' their hands before entering.

'Bacteria are particularly scared of white plastic pinnies!' Dr Fraser told us, smiling wryly as he pulled his white pinny over his head.

One of the constraints of being neutropenic is that you can't eat any raw fruit or vegetables. Coupled with the fact that Rachel's mouth was full of ulcers and that she was regularly hit by waves of nausea, meal times became an onerous chore.

'I've got to make myself eat' she would say 'otherwise how am I going to have the energy to fight this?'

However, this was easier said than done. Despite Nick's readiness to wolf down the Australian hospital tucker, the food that appeared on her table was far from appetising. Even so, she would always make a valiant attempt at it, until one Saturday morning. She had carefully selected a jacket potato and cottage cheese for lunch.

'The inside of the potato is quite soft and the cheese quite bland, so it won't hurt my mouth' she rationalised.

Lunchtime came and a warm, covered plate arrived. I lifted the plastic covering to reveal a heap of lukewarm cottage cheese and some fast wilting salad. Rachel looked incredulous.

'I can't eat that' she told a somewhat bewildered orderly, 'it's got salad on it, I can't have salad ... there is no potato and I can't even touch the cheese because it's next to the salad.'

'She is neutropenic' I qualified, stupidly, as I realised the poor orderly had no idea why we were making a fuss. After all she did not prepare the food and had no idea what neutropenic meant.

'All potatoes eaten ... no left ... all gone eaten today' she explained in broken English.

Rachel decided she'd wait until dinner to eat, her appetite was not too great at that time anyway. But, she was adamant she was not going to stand for such poor nutritional care. She asked the staff nurse for the catering manager's number and phoned her to complain about the standard of food given her special dietary needs.

'I'm not fussy' she emphasised, 'but I wasn't able to touch anything on the plate.'

She was assured that this would not happen again. It was true – it didn't, in fact nothing happened! Dinner came and went, as did breakfast the next morning, with no food appearing at all. The next morning I arrived back at the hospital to find Rachel upset and indignant. She had had no food since the lunch she couldn't touch and was rightly feeling neglected and hungry. The nursing staff had contacted the catering department but to no avail. The catering manager eventually made an appearance in Rachel's room (adorned with the mandatory white apron) on Tuesday afternoon to discuss her dietary requirements. In the meantime she had survived on Morwenna's chicken soup which we froze in bags and defrosted for her. Interestingly this episode was the catalyst for an examination of the communication channels between the catering department, dieticians and the rest of the multi-professional team.

Being neutropenic was difficult for another reason that summer. Some of our friends had started to get married and Rachel was missing their summer weddings. This was not on as far as she was concerned! So, on one occasion, having monitored her white cell count all week she discharged herself on a Saturday to attend a friend's wedding on a boat on the Thames. She returned to the ward on the Sunday exhausted but triumphant. Jubilant at having broken out of the 'patient' role even though it was just for an evening.

During her treatment her main interest was understandably whether the size of her tumour was reducing. Early on in the course of her second run of chemotherapy, a date was set for a scan and the subsequent comparison of the treatment results with a pre-chemotherapy scan. Dr Fraser was not available and his senior registrar, Dr Phillips, was conducting the consultation. Upon reflection, we did not put him in a very easy situation. When he arrived at lunchtime, four of Rachel's friends (one a doctor herself) and myself were sitting in her hospital room, desperate to hear that the treatment had been a success. We piled into the consulting room and looked at the two lit scans that were pinned on the wall.

'Well' he began, 'this is the initial scan and here you can see the tumour.'

He indicated a large, dark mass, 'and as you can see on the second scan, it hasn't really reduced much in size, so I would say that the chemotherapy isn't really working.'

He talked at the scan, glancing sporadically at his feet. There was a stunned silence.

'So what are you saying ... what should I do? ... there must be something else you can do' Rachel was desperate. We bombarded him with questions. Was he sure? What were the alternatives?

'If it was me, I'd keep going' Dr Phillips paused and looked at his feet again, 'but that's me. It doesn't seem like there will be much success.'

It didn't seem to make sense. Then, in the silence, Sally, Rachel's doctor friend, pointed out,

'You're comparing a CAT scan with an MRI scan.' The pre-chemotherapy scan was not the same type as the more recent scan! The task of interpreting the two scans was quickly handed onto Dr Fraser who was currently away at a conference. Waiting for a possible death sentence left Rachel in anguish for a couple of days. However, this time Dr Fraser's interpretation of the scans actually resulted in a decision to continue treatment.

Throughout 1997 and 1998 she continued to battle her way through the British healthcare system, at some times carried by caring health professionals and at others left confused and bewildered by the less competent. Throughout her treatment she valiantly shied away from the 'patient role', constantly seeking information about new and alternative treatments which may increase her chance of life, desperate to maintain a sense of control. The harsh reality was in fact that the cancer was fast becoming the controller.

In May 1998, following a period of remission during which Rachel had been enjoying paragliding, holidaying in South Africa and hiking in the Peak District, she had another follow-up appointment with Dr Fraser. The previous week she had had a number of tests and scans. She still found the scanning experience isolating and frightening, but luckily could always find a male friend to accompany her and hold her hand. She was sure they quite fancied a particularly pretty nurse! On the Friday of the appointment our father drove us to the hospital. I had arranged to go to Dublin for the weekend with some university friends, and had slung my weekend bag into the boot. 'If it's good news I'll go straight to the airport – and if not – well Dublin can wait' was my rationale. We sat waiting for what seemed like an eternity in a small waiting room with 1970s style posters promoting the benefits of regular exercise hanging limply from the wall. Dr Fraser had been caught up at the private hospital where he had had a clinic that morning and was now stuck in traffic, a nurse told us. The waiting and not knowing when he would arrive made every minute seem like a day. Dad had brought some work with him, but was obviously not concentrating on it at all. Eventually the same nurse ushered us into the office of an apologetic Dr Fraser, who told us that he had not been able to get the blood results and was just going to take a look at the scans.

'Shall I phone the lab and ask them to fax the blood results through to you, or call your PA?' I asked, surprising myself and Dr Fraser. Having worked in a not dissimilar Australian health service I was acutely aware of the need to be proactive to make things happen. I was also determined that we were not going to go away and come back next week just because some results hadn't been faxed over in time.

'Oh ... why not, OK, thanks' Dr Fraser indicated to a phone in the corner 'it's extension 475, tell them that Dr Fraser needs them within the next three minutes.' He disappeared off to retrieve the scans.

It was clear upon his return that all was not well. The tumour had returned, he told us, and the only option was surgery that would in essence be palliative. He directed this information awkwardly at our father. His own daughters were little younger than Rachel and myself and he was clearly acutely aware of what our father was feeling. Rachel battled to take stock of the information she had heard, grasping at straws.

'But it might work, mightn't it?'

The question hung unanswered in the air.

Shortly after this she was ushered off by a nurse to soak her arms in a basin of warm water, so that a junior doctor could take some blood from her battered veins for potential future transfusions. It was hard for the junior doctor to find a vein. After three failed attempts, I asked,

'Can't you take my blood, it's exactly the same, we're genetically the same.' Obviously not, a second question remained unanswered and the junior doctor looked at me as if I was slightly mad.

Dublin could wait. Rachel decided to go out with some friends that night for dinner, to try to find some normality and forget the awfulness of that afternoon. After a quiet dinner with Angus (now my husband to be), I was sound asleep when the phone rang just after 2.00am. There was no voice, just hysterical gasping and sobbing.

'Stay there' I said 'I'll be two minutes.'

We tore down the stairs of the flat, me still in my pyjamas. We jumped in the car and drove frantically to Rachel's house, luckily only a few roads away. She literally fell out of the doorway into our arms sobbing, shaking and crying. There is nothing as desperately isolating and deeply sad as the thoughts and fears of a 27-year-old girl facing her own death, alone in the middle of the night. We wrapped her up in a duvet and took her home. But this surface security couldn't touch the turmoil of fear of pain, dying and death that was going on inside. The next day we located the local out-of-hours GP service. For once Rachel was feeling too fragile to negotiate treatment for herself and the task of obtaining a prescription for sleeping tablets to give her some brief respite was left to Angus (a trainee doctor at the time).

For me, one of the most poignant of the many memories I have of those days is of Rachel lying in a hospital bed after her final operation, intended principally to reduce the intense pressure and pain within her sinuses. Her face was once again swollen, her hair short and eyebrows still re-growing. I sat by her bed whilst she talked sporadically, slipping in and out of morphine-induced sleep. She spoke coherently sometimes, then lapsed into stories of her 'cats running triathlons'! The morphine speaking. In the midst of this her current pain consultant arrived. Immediately she was alert, forcing her mind clear of its morphine-induced fog. The consultant glanced at me and smiled. 'This is my twin sister' she said, 'my twin.' She turned her head towards the nursing sister standing beside the consultant, checking she had understood.

What was so deeply moving, indeed heart wrenching, was the true meaning behind what she was trying to communicate ... 'I am a normal person – this is what I am meant to look like, a healthy, strong young woman.' Yet her puffy face, her scarred body and

medical records combined to deny this fact. Pure and unjust disso-
nance.

In July 1998, we drove across London, to meet with Dr Fraser at a
private hospital north of the river. Desperate to be in control, Rachel
gave Angus somewhat dubious directions, as she was distracted and
anxious about the pending consultation. We didn't wait long at all
this time. Dr Fraser welcomed us into his consulting room and
attached a 'do not disturb' sign to the outside of the door.

'Rachel, I am afraid the tumour has returned and it is growing.'
Silence.

'Isn't there anything else you can do?' She was struggling to stay
calm.

'Not without you losing the sight in both eyes, you see it's very
close to the optic chiasma.' At this point Dr Fraser scribbled a very
messy diagram of the optic nerves on the back of a letter on his
desk. As an ex-biology teacher I would certainly have asked for this
to be re-done if it had been submitted as homework by a pupil! He
then went into a technical description of how the optic nerves are
connected and how vision is affected by the structure of the eye.
Rachel clearly was taking none of this in.

'So am I going to go blind? Am I going to die? Isn't there anything
you can do? What about this new laser treatment?'

The technical description continued with Angus awkwardly trying
to explain what Dr Fraser was saying in layman's terms.

'I don't want to live if I go blind ... but there must be something
else ... the laser treatment.' Rachel was desperate for him to throw
her a lifeline and he was finding it difficult to tell a beautiful young
woman that she was going to die. He was hinting at it and she in
turn was resisting the message.

'I don't know much about the laser treatment Rachel, but I know
a lady who does, Dr X ... look', he ferreted around in the piles of
paper on his desk and fished out a photo, 'this is a picture of us
drinking cappuccino together in a café in Amsterdam ... we were at
a conference there in March.'

'Dr Fraser' I was desperate for some clarity, 'if Rachel was your
daughter, what would you want her to take away from this consultation?'

He put the photo down and looked at Rachel.

'That there is nothing else I can do.'

Earlier in the year Rachel had bought herself a little flat in Putney,
London, longing for security, stability and her own space. Yet as the
cancer tightened its grip, the foundations of her world were rocked
so strongly that no bricks and mortar could protect her. Her flat

became a haven from the world. It was constantly filled with cards and flowers, but was also awash with bottles of medication, vials and syringes. There had been no 'seamless care' when she was discharged from hospital for the last time. She arrived home to a flat on her own and struggled with the basic daily chores of shopping, eating and washing her clothes. By chance we discovered that she was entitled to social services help and arranged for Lorna, a wonderful Jamaican home help, to come in every other day to clean, shop and sing (an added extra). The district nurse made a couple of visits but was confused by the multitude of drugs Rachel had to take throughout the day. She left Rachel who was intelligent but ill, not medical and equally confused, a pill tray labelled with the days of the weeks and times of the day. Angus and Rachel spent an afternoon sorting out the drugs and putting them into the right compartments. An invaluable experience for a trainee doctor.

Although surrounded by family and friends she was so alone, isolated by her disease and the creeping realisation of her own mortality. Her diary, whilst still full, detailed medical appointments rather than dinner dates, and as time passed the 'hospital' appointments morphed into 'hospice' appointments.

The hospice gradually became a greater part of Rachel's life. To start, the idea of a hospice appalled her. Visiting the hospice would be like giving in to death. Her Macmillan nurse, a wonderfully sensitive and empathic person, encouraged Rachel to visit the hospice.

'Just for a morning. So that if you ever need a break you can pop over there and you'll know where to go.'

Her visit started with a massage from the hospice therapist, and later a talk with the chaplain. She began to spend mornings over at the hospice, talking about the experiences she was facing ... her thoughts moving farther away from those that concern most 28-year-olds. In a strange way she became empowered again, and certainly touched by the gentleness and calm of the place.

In the last week of November I arrived at Rachel's flat on a Sunday morning, somewhat jaded. It was the night after my hen night. We sat eating rice pudding for breakfast, one of the only foods her ulcer ridden mouth could palate.

'There is something wrong with my eye' she said. She had already lost the sight in her left eye.

'It looks OK to me Rach.'

'It's not' she was firm, 'it's just the same as with my other eye. I need to see someone about it. What if I go blind?'

It was Sunday, where was I going to find an ophthalmic specialist, if that was what I needed? Would they know about rhabdomyosarcomas? After three lengthy phone calls with the hospital we located a specialist who was working in London that afternoon. If we drove over to see him at 4.00pm he may be able to help. At 3.45pm we were sitting in a draughty corridor of a Victorian building. A harassed looking nurse appeared briefly, asked us who we had come to see and disappeared without a word! Did the consultant know we were here? 5.00pm came and then 5.30pm – I went to find a nurse (equally harassed but a different one this time).

'I think there is a doctor coming, I am not sure.'

'Could you find out for us please?' She agreed that she probably could.

Shortly after 6.00 an exhausted registrar arrived. She took a look at Rachel's eye and was, she said, out of her depth.

'I don't know, this isn't really my area. You'll need to come back tomorrow and see the consultant. I think he has a clinic on Monday or Tuesday. But don't worry' she added, 'If you get a 7th nerve palsy on this side we can always stitch your eyelid open.'

'What if something gets into my eye?' Rachel asked on the way home, her anxiety heightened rather than allayed.

Friday 28 November 1998, 11.00am. My mobile rings, strange I hardly ever turn it on. I am at a meeting at a hospital in Sussex.

'Hello, is that Naomi? It's Helen here, one of the nurses at the hospice' I distinctly remember a soft, steady, Irish voice.

'I've got Rachel here with me' my skin prickled. 'She'd like some company, how soon can you get here?'

Soon. I ran to the car and negotiated my way through the congested roads to London. I reached the hospice and abandoned my car in the front car park. I half ran, half walked to the ward, sensing the calm of the place – a complete contrast to my own feelings, aware that I had to be calm myself.

'Hello love' Helen again. 'You must be Naomi, you two are very similar.' Rachel would have been pleased to hear this. 'Would you like to come into the nurses' office so I can just tell you how she is doing?'

I let myself be led.

'Lorna found her collapsed in the bathroom this morning, she has lost the sight in her other eye and is very poorly so we brought her in here by ambulance. I don't think she'll make the weekend. I'm sorry.' She looked directly at me as she spoke and put her hand out to touch my arm. 'Do you want some time before you go in and see her?'

No, I just wanted to be with her.

'Hello Rach' I crept in and held her hand. Helen stood quietly just by the door, checking we were both OK. 'It's me.'

'Hello me' she spoke slowly. 'I don't think I am going to make it to your wedding.' She was due to be our bridesmaid in two weeks' time.

Rachel spent five days in the hospice, visited by a multitude of friends and family. The nursing staff never tired of repeating updates on Rachel's health to the many enquirers. Dr Craig, the palliative care consultant, made unlimited time for the family. She took Nick and I into the relatives room, explaining what was happening to Rachel and giving us the chance to ask as many questions as we wanted (she repeated the same exercise for our parents and our natural mother Elaine). Assuring us that she would experience no pain. She was right. It was interesting to watch her interact with Rachel. Even at the end when it was unclear as to how much Rachel was conscious of, she looked at her face when she talked, held her hand and talked to her as an equal, a behaviour mirrored by the nursing staff. It was also wonderful and refreshing, as a relative, to be included in the care, involved in the decision making and cared for as an integral part of the dying experience.

Rachel died peacefully in the early hours of 2 December 1998, aged twenty-eight and a half.

Towards the end of her illness I heard a friend saying to Rachel 'You are so brave, the way you are dealing with your cancer.' She had replied 'I'm not brave, I don't have a choice.' I would argue that her friend was right, she was brave, brave enough to write her story, to revisit what were undoubtedly the most difficult times of her life, and to share these with the world in order that others may learn from her experiences. Her account is a legacy, rich not only in her detailed descriptions of the experience of living with cancer, but also, importantly, in her psychologist's unravelling of what health professionals can learn from her story.

If there was ever a story that deserved telling, it is this. But what Rachel would have wished most dearly is that her story be listened to – and acted upon.

References

1   Molleman E (1984) The significance of the doctor-patient relationship in coping with cancer. *Soc Sci Med.* **18**: 475–80.

2   Chaitchik S, Kreitler S, Shaked S, *et al.* Doctor-patient communication in a cancer ward. Source unknown.

3   Guex P. *An Introduction to Psycho-oncology.* Trans Heather Goodare.

4   Anderson BL (1992) Psychological interventions for cancer patients to enhance the quality of life. *J Consult Clin Psychol.* **60**: 552–68.

5   Silverman D (1987) *Communication and Medical Practice: social relations in the clinic.* Sage, London.

6   Buckman L (1984) Breaking bad news: why is it still so difficult? *BMJ.* **2**: 1623–7.

7   Bloch R. Disclosing cancer diagnosis to a patient. *J Nat Cancer Inst.* **86**: 868.

8   Fallowfield L (1993) Giving sad and bad news. *Lancet.* **341**: 467–8.

9   Cassileth BR and Steinfeld AD (1987) Psychological preparation of the patient and family. *Cancer.* **60**: 547–52.

10 Maguire P and Faulkner A (1988) Communicating with cancer patients: 1 Handling bad news and difficult questions. *BMJ.* **297**: 907–9.

11 Maguire P and Faulkner A (1988) Communicating with cancer patients: 2 Handling uncertainty, collusion and denial. *BMJ.* **297**: 972–4.

12 Sardell A and Trieweiler S (1993) Disclosing the cancer diagnosis. *Cancer.* **72**: 3355–65.

13 Butow P, Kazeim J, Beeney L, *et al.* (1996) When the diagnosis is cancer. *American Cancer Journal.* 2630–37.

14 Buller MK and Buller DB (1987) Physicians' communication style and patient satisfaction. *J Health Soc Behav.* **28**: 375–88.

15 Bartlett EE, Grayson M, Barker R, *et al.* (1984) The effects of physician communication skills on patient satisfaction, recall and adherance. *J Chronic Dis.* **37**: 755–64.

16 Bertakis K, Roter D and Putman S. The relationship of physician medical interview style to patient satisfaction. Source unknown.

17 Sell L, Devlin B, Bourke SJ, *et al.* (1993) Communicating the diagnosis of lung cancer. *Respir Med.* **87**: 61–3.

18   Lind SE, Good MD, Seidel S, *et al.* (1993) Telling the diagnosis of cancer. *J Clin Oncol.* **7**(5): 583–9.

19   Tattersal MHN, Butow PN, Griffin AM, *et al.* The take home message. Patients prefer consultation audiotapes to summary letters. Personal communication.

20   Ford S, Fallowfield L and Lewis S (1994) Can oncologists detect distress in their out-patients and how satisified are they with their performance during bad news consultations? *Br J Cancer.* **70**: 767–70.

21   Paraskevaidis E, Kitchener HC and Walker LG (1993) Doctor-patient communication and subsequent mental health in women with gynae-cological cancer. *Psycho-oncology.* **2**: 195–200.

22   Selvin ML (1987) Talking about cancer: how much is too much? *Br J Hosp Med.* **38**: 56–9.

23   Greer and Watson (1987) Mental adjustment to cancer: its measure-ment and prognostic importance. *Cancer Surveys.* **6**: 439–53.

24   Dunn SM, Patterson PU, Butow PN, *et al.* (1993) Cancer by another name: a randomised trial of the effects of euphemism and uncertainty in communicating with patients. *J Clin Oncol.* **11**: 989–96.

25   Butow PN, Dunn SM, Tattersal MHN, *et al.* (1994) Patient participa-tion in the cancer consultation: evaluation of a question prompt sheet. *Ann Oncol.* **5**: 199–204.

26   Maguire P (1992) Improving the recognition and treatment of affective disorders in cancer patients. *Recent Adv Psychiatry.* **7**: 15–30.

27   Burish TG, Snyder SL and Jenkins RA (2001) Preparing patients for chemotherapy: effects of coping preparation and relaxation interven-tion. *J Consult Clin Psychol.* **59**: 518–25.

28   North N, Cornbleet MA, Knowles G, Leonard RCF. Information giving in oncology: a preliminary study of tape-recorder use. *Br J Clin Psychol.* **31**: 357–9.

29   Sutherland H, Llewelyn-Thomas H, Lockwood G, *et al.* (1989) Cancer patients: their desire for information and participation in treatment decisions. *J Roy Soc Med.* **82**: 260–4.

30   Fallowfield L and Clark A (1991) *Breast Cancer.* Routledge, London.

31   Grossath-Maticek R and Eysenk H (1988) Length of survival and lymphocyte percentage in women with mammary cancer as a function of psychotherapy. *Psychol Rep.* **65**: 315–21.

32   Faulkner A, Pearce G and O'Keefe C (1995) *When a Child has Cancer.* Chapman & Hall, London.

33   Wiley C and Sillman RA. The impact of disease on the social support experiences of cancer patients. *Psychosoc Oncol.* **8**(1): 79–96.

34   Buller MK and Buller DB (1987) Physicians' communication style and patient satisfaction. *J Health and Soc Behav.* **28**: 375–88.

35   Lind SE, Good MD, Seidel S, *et al.* (1993) Telling the diagnosis of cancer. *J Clin Oncol.* **7**(5): 583–9.

36   Cohen SR, Mount BM, Tomas JJN, *et al.* (1996) Existential well-being is an important determinant of quality of life. *Cancer.* **77**: 576–86.

37   Dean C and Surtees PG. Do psychological factors predict survival in breast cancer? *J Psychosom Res.* **33**: 561–9.

38   Ratcliffe MA, Dawson AA and Walker LG (1995) Eysenk personality L-scores in patients with Hodgkin's disease and non-Hodgkin's lymphoma. *Psycho-oncology.* **4**: 39–45.

39   Spiegal D, Bloom JR, Kramer HC, *et al.* (1989) Effects of psychosocial treatment on the survival of patients with metastatic breast cancer. *Lancet.* **ii**: 888–91.

40   Bloom JR, Hayes WA, Saunders F, *et al.* (1987) Cancer awareness and secondary prevention practices in black Americans: implications for intervention. *Family and Community Health.* **10**: 19–30.

41   Cassileth BR, Lusk EJ, Miller DS, *et al.* (1985) Psychosocial correlation of survival in advanced malignant disease. *New Engl J Med.* **312**(24): 1551–73.

42   Cassileth BR, Walsh WP and Lusk EJ. Psychological correlation of cancer survival: a subsequent report 3 to 8 years after cancer diagnosis. *J Clin Oncol.* **6**(11): 1753–9.

43   Bloom JR, Kang SH and Romano P (1991) *Cancer and Stress: the effect of social support as a resource. Cancer and Stress: psychological, biological and coping studies.* John Wiley, Chichester.

44   Goodwin JS, Hunt WC, Key CR, *et al.* (1987) The effects of marital status on stage, treatment and survival of cancer patients. *JAMA.* **258**: 3125–30.

45   Neale AV, Tidley BC and Vernon SW. Marital status: delay in seeking treatment and survival from breast cancer. *Soc Sci Med.* **23**: 305–12.

46   Moorey S. The psychological impact of cancer. In: P Webb (ed.) *Oncology for Nurses and Health Care Professionals.* Harper & Row, London.

47   Walker LG and Eremin O (1996) Psychological assessment and intervention: future prospects for women with breast cancer. *Semin Surg Oncol.* **12**: 76–83.

48   Maguire P. Barriers to psychological care of the dying. *BMJ.* **291**: 1711–13.

49   Massie MJ and Holland JC. Overview of normal reaction and prevalence of psychiatric disorders. In: JC Holland and JH Rowland (eds) *Handbook of Psycho-oncology.* Oxford University Press, New York.

50   Maguire P. Improving the detection of psychiatric problems in cancer patients. *Soc Sci Med.* **20**: 819–23.

51   Fox BH (1989) Depressive symptoms and the risk of cancer. *JAMA.* **262**(9): 1231.

52   Pettingale KW, Morris T, Greer S, *et al.* (1985) Mental attitudes to cancer: an additional prognostic factor. *Lancet.* **i**: 50.

53   Levy SM and Wise BD. Psychosocial risk factors in cancer prognosis. In: CR Cooper (ed.) *Stress and Breast Cancer.* John Wiley, Chichester.

54   Mahrer AR (1980) The treatment of cancer through experiential psychotherapy. *Psychother Theor Res Prac.* **17**: 335–42.

55   Luce JK and Dawson JJ (1975) Quality of life. *Semin Oncol.* **2**: 323–7.

56 Weismann A, Worden W and Sorbel H. *Project Omega: psychosocial screening and intervention with cancer patients.* Source unknown.

57 Gordon WA, Friedenbergs I, Diller L, *et al.* (1980) Efficacy of psychosocial intervention with cancer patients. *J Consul Clin Psychol.* **48**: 743–59.

58 Forester B, Kornfeld D and Fleiss J (1985) Psychotherapy during radiotherapy: effects on emotional and physical distress. *Am J Psychol.* **142**(1): 22–7.

59 Spiegal D and Glafkides M (1983) Effects of group confrontation with death and dying. *Int J Psychoter.* **33**(4): 433–47.

60 Galinsky MJ (1985) Groups for cancer patients and their families: purposes and group conditions. In: M Sundel, P Glasser, R Sarri and R Venter (eds) *Individual Change Through Small Groups* (2e). Free Press, New York.

61 Telch CF and Telch MJ (1985) Psychological approaches to enhancing coping among cancer patients: a review. *Clin Psychol Review.* **5**: 325–44.

62 Telch CF and Telch MJ (1986) Group coping skills instruction and supportive group therapy for cancer patients: a comparison of strategies. *J Consult Clin Psychol.* **54**(6): 802–8.

63 Morrow GR and Morrell L (1982) Behaviour treatment for the anticipatory nausea induced by cancer chemotherapy. *New Eng J Med.* **307**: 1476–80.

64 Lyles JN, Burish TG, Krozley MG, *et al.* (1982) Efficacy of relaxation training and guided imagery in reducing the aversiveness of cancer chemotherapy. *J Consult Clin Psychol.* **50**: 509–24.

65 Tarrier N and Maguire GP (1984) Treatment of psychological distress following mastectomy: an initial report. *Behav Res Ther.* **22**: 81–4.

66 Hopwood P and Maguire GP (1988) Body image problems in cancer patients. *Br J Psych.* **153**(2): 47–50.

67 Moorey S and Greer S (1989) Adjuvant psychological therapy: a cognitive behavioural treatment for patients with cancer. *Behav Psychother.* **17**: 177–90.

68 Greer S and Moorey S (1990) Evaluation of adjunct psychological therapy for clinically referred cancer patients. *Brit J Can.*

69 Maguire P, Hopwood P, Tarrier N, *et al.* (1985) Treatment of depression in cancer patients. *Acta Psych Scand.* **72**(320): 81–4.

70 Grossath-Maticek R, Schmidt P, Vetter N, *et al.* (1984) Psychotherapy research in oncology. In: A Steptoe and S Mathew (eds) *Health Care and Human Behaviour.* Academic Press, London.

71 Bagenal FS, Easton DF, Harris E, *et al.* (1990) Survival of patients with breast cancer attending Bristol Cancer Help Centre. *Lancet.* **336**: 606–10.

72 Watson M and Ramirez A (1991) Psychological factors in cancer prognosis. In: *Cancer and Stress: psychological, biological and coping studies.* John Wiley, Chichester.

73 Fawzy FI, Fawzy NW, Hyun CS, *et al.* (1993) Malignant melanoma: effects of an early structured psychiatric intervention, coping and affective state on recurrence and survival 5 years later. *Arch Gen Psychiatry.* **50**: 621–89.

74 Holland JC and Rowland JH (eds) (1989) *Handbook of Psycho-oncology: psychological care of the patient with cancer.* Oxford University Press, Oxford.

75 Pendleton D, Schofield T, Tate P, *et al.* (1984) *The Consultation: an approach to teaching and learning.* GP Series No. 6. Oxford University Press, Oxford.

76 Pendleton D, Schofield T, Tate P, *et al.* (2001) *The Consultation: an approach to teaching and learning* (2e). Oxford University Press, Oxford.

77 Byrne PS and Long BEL (1976) *Doctors Talking to Patients.* HMSO, London.

78 Salinsky J and Sackin P (2000) *What Are You Feeling, Doctor? Identifying and avoiding defensive patterns in the consultation.* Radcliffe Medical Press, Oxford.

Index